£32.50

5/12/2005

NLM
Class
Mark:
L.G.I.

WL
356
LOS

D1336461

# Neurological Rehabilitation of Stroke

The Queen Square Rehabilitation Series

# Neurological Rehabilitation of Stroke

*Edited by*
**Nick Losseff MD FRCP**

*Consultant Neurologist*
*The National Hospital for Neurology and Neurosurgery*
*University College London Hospitals Trust*
*and The Whittington Hospital*
*London, UK*

*Series Editor*
**Alan J Thompson MD FRCP FRCPI**

*Garfield Weston Professor*
*of Clinical Neurology and Neurorehabilitation*
*Institute of Neurology, University College London*
*and Clinical Director and Hononary Consultant in Neurology*
*The National Hospital for Neurology and Neurosurgery*
*University College London Hospitals Trust*
*Queen Square, London, UK*

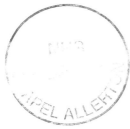

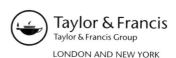

Taylor & Francis
Taylor & Francis Group

LONDON AND NEW YORK

A MARTIN DUNITZ BOOK

© 2004 Taylor & Francis, an imprint of the Taylor & Francis Group

First published in the United Kingdom in 2004
by Taylor & Francis, an imprint of the Taylor & Francis Group, 11 New Fetter Lane,
London EC4P 4EE

Tel.:        +44 (0) 20 7583 9855
Fax.:       +44 (0) 20 7842 2298
E-mail:    info@dunitz.co.uk
Website:  http://www.dunitz.co.uk

All rights reserved. No part of this publication may be reproduced, stored in a
retrieval system, or transmitted, in any form or by any means, electronic, mechanical,
photocopying, recording, or otherwise, without the prior permission of the publisher
or in accordance with the provisions of the Copyright, Designs and Patents Act 1988
or under the terms of any licence permitting limited copying issued by the Copyright
Licensing Agency, 90 Tottenham Court Road, London W1P 0LP.

Although every effort has been made to ensure that all owners of copyright material
have been acknowledged in this publication, we would be glad to acknowledge in
subsequent reprints or editions any omissions brought to our attention.

A CIP record for this book is available from the British Library.

Library of Congress Cataloging-in-Publication Data

Data available on application

ISBN 1-84184-322-9

Distributed in North and South America by
Taylor & Francis
2000 NW Corporate Blvd
Boca Raton, FL 33431, USA

*Within Continental USA*
Tel.: 800 272 7737; Fax: 800 374 3401
*Outside Continental USA*
Tel.: 561 994 0555; Fax: 561 361 6018
E-mail: orders@crcpress.com

Distributed in the rest of the world by
Thomson Publishing Services
Cheriton House
North Way
Andover, Hampshire SP10 5BE, UK
Tel.: +44 (0)1264 332424
E-mail: salesorder.tandf@thomsonpublishingservices.co.uk

Composition by Peter Powell Origination & Print Limited, Maidstone, Kent
Printed and bound in Great Britain by The Cromwell Press Ltd, Trowbridge, Wilts.

# Contents

# Contributors

**Helena Bryant**
Occupational Therapist
The Acute Brain Injury Unit
The National Hospital for
    Neurology and Neurosurgery
Queen Square
London, UK

**Linsey Clarke**
Speech and Language Therapist
The Acute Brain Injury Unit
The National Hospital for
    Neurology and Neurosurgery
Queen Square
London, UK

**Richard Greenwood**
Consultant Neurologist
Acute Brain Injury Service
The National Hospital for
    Neurology and Neurosurgery,
and Regional Neurological
    Rehabilitation Unit
Homerton Hospital
London, UK

**Sarah Guy**
Physiotherapist
The Acute Brain Injury Unit
The National Hospital for
    Neurology and Neurosurgery
Queen Square
London, UK

**Robert McCrum**
Literary Editor to *The Observer*

**Lalit Kalra**
Professor of Stroke Medicine
Department of Diabetes,
    Endocrinology and Internal
    Medicine
Guy's, King's & St Thomas'
    School of Medicine
Denmark Hill Campus
Bessemer Road
London, UK

**Nick Losseff**
Consultant Neurologist
The National Hospital for
    Neurology and Neurosurgery
UCL Hospitals Trust, London
    and The Whittington
    Hospital, London
Honorary Senior Lecturer in
    Neurology
University College London
London, UK

**Mehool Patel**
Consultant Physician in Stroke
    & Elderly Medicine
University Hospital Lewisham
Guy's, King's and St Thomas'
    School of Medicine
King's College
London, UK

**Gail Robinson**
Neuropsychologist
The Acute Brain Injury Unit
The National Hospital for
    Neurology and Neurosurgery
Queen Square
London, UK

**Anthony Rudd**
Consultant in Stroke Medicine
Director, RCP Working Party
    on Stroke
St Thomas's Hospital
Guy's, King's and St Thomas'
    School of Medicine
King's College
London, UK

**Ella Segaran**
Dietician
The Acute Brain Injury Unit
The National Hospital for
    Neurology and Neurosurgery
Queen Square
London, UK

**Trudy Stewart**
Ward Manager
The Acute Brain Injury Unit
The National Hospital for
    Neurology and Neurosurgery
Queen Square
London, UK

**Nick S Ward**
Consultant Neurologist
Wellcome Department of
    Imaging Neuroscience
Institute of Neurology
University College London
The National Hospital for
    Neurology and Neurosurgery
Queen Square
London, UK

# Series Preface

Neurological rehabilitation aims to lessen the impact of neurological disorders and maximize their impact on those affected by them. The importance of managing the consequences of acute and chronic neurological disorders is increasingly acknowledged, as is the role that neurologists can and should play in minimizing their impact. This has required a broader focus for neurological practice, which, in turn, has a major implication for training.

This series, written by people from a variety of backgrounds, is an attempt to deliver the essentials of neurological rehabilitation in a concise and user-friendly fashion. It will cover a range of neurological disorders, all of which have a major impact on those affected. The second in the series aims to provide an evidence base for stroke rehabilitation. It brings together a multidisciplinary team of experts and is edited by Dr Nick Losseff. It is hoped that by publishing the essential elements in a concise and accessible format it will prove a useful and much used aid in patient management.

*Alan J Thompson*
*Series Editor*

# Preface

This book aims to provide the reader with an evidence base for stroke rehabilitation and, along with the other titles in the series, it has followed a specific formula. First we have explored the molecular basis of neural recovery and restoration following vascular injury, then illustrated the practical aspects of interdisciplinary working in an acute environment, the population-based impact of stroke, the tools of outcome assessment and finally models of service delivery.

We have been very fortunate to assemble leading figures within these fields for all chapters and in particular thank Robert McCrum for his personal view, which should be read by all professionals involved in stroke care.

The management of stroke is entering a renaissance; partly in the UK due to central recognition of the tremendous public health problem it poses. Thus new services are developing in parallel with significant advances in acute treatments and increased understanding of the mechanisms of neural recovery and restoration. Stroke provides the ideal model by which 'acute' treatment and 'rehabilitation' can be seen as a continuum. We hope this book will be of use to all professionals involved in the care of patients with stroke.

*Nick Losseff*

# The Potential for Recovery and Repair Following Stroke

*Nick S Ward*

Work in both animals and humans suggests that the brain is not hard-wired. The notion that the brain, and in particular the cortex, has the capacity to change structure and consequently function is now widely accepted. In addition the lesioned brain may have greater potential to undergo these plastic changes than the normal brain. Rehabilitative training appears to be a vital component needed to facilitate these changes.

## Introduction

Patients suffering from a stroke often undergo some degree of functional recovery (Twitchell, 1951). The extent of this recovery, to some degree, can be predicted on the basis of parameters such as lesion size, premorbid health, etc. However, significant variation occurs, implying that outcome is influenced by many variables. It is the responsibility of the clinician to attempt to influence these variables so as to facilitate the best possible outcome for each patient. To date the cornerstone of restorative neurology in the field of stroke has comprised supportive medical care and more specific therapies (physiotherapy, occupational therapy, speech and language therapy). However, clinicians are becoming aware of advances made in the basic sciences, which will add a new dimension to the treatment of functional deficits in patients suffering stroke and other single insult brain injuries.

## The Basis of Stroke Management

In the first few minutes and hours after stroke, physicians take an active approach to management, with the aim of preserving as much brain tissue as possible (Brown, 2002). Thrombolytic therapy using tissue plasminogen activator is beneficial in acute ischaemic stroke, but only when given within 3 hours of onset, to suitable patients in specialized units (Lees, 2000).

Many neuroprotective drugs have been tested successfully in animal models of stroke, but none has proved effective in randomized trials in man. However, other non-pharmacological strategies are often employed to protect the brain from further ischaemia and extension of infarction. For example, systolic blood pressure can be maintained within a given range, antipyretic drugs given for fever and blood glucose maintained within the normal range. Nevertheless, despite these measures many patients with stroke continue to have significant disability after the acute period. Hence, enhancing recovery using modern rehabilitation techniques continues to play an essential part in stroke treatment.

Randomized clinical trials have provided good evidence that the best way to enhance recovery is to admit the patient to a stroke unit (Stroke Unit Trialists' Collaboration, 1997, 2000). These benefits are achieved not simply by gathering the patients together in a single location labelled 'stroke unit', but by the development of a specialized multidisciplinary team who have ownership of the complex problems experienced by patients. How much each component contributes to the success of the stroke unit is not entirely clear, but recent evidence supports the effectiveness of physiotherapy for stroke patients in the post-acute phase. A meta-analysis combining results of seven randomized controlled trials on the effects of different intensities of therapy after stroke reported small but significant reductions in mortality and significant improvements in activities of daily living (ADL) scores as a result of higher intensity therapy (Langhorne et al, 1996). Furthermore, Kwakkel et al (1997) examined nine trials of physiotherapy in stroke patients involving 1051 patients, and concluded that there was a small but significant correlation between intensity of therapy and outcome. In addition, targeted therapy may have a specific rather than non-specific effect, e.g. greater intensity of leg rehabilitation improves functional recovery and health-related functional status, whereas greater intensity of arm rehabilitation results in small improvements in hand dexterity (Kwakkel et al, 1999). This suggests that failure to demonstrate a benefit with physiotherapy in the past might be related to the fact that assessments were often made using global ADL scales, rather than parameters relating directly to the form of training being given. For example, a study involving 148 hemiparetic patients undergoing an intensive period of training, demonstrated that gait symmetry (a principle goal of many physiotherapy programmes) was unaffected. However, specific measurements of stance duration, weight acceptance, and push off of both legs improved significantly (Hesse et al, 1994). Furthermore, recovery of gait function in the severely hemiplegic patient using treadmill training, functional electrical stimulation, individually or in combination with each other, has been demonstrated to improve specific aspects of gait, indicating a significant task-specific training effect (Hesse et al, 1995).

It might be argued that the only truly *relevant* measurements are global functional assessments in the home environment. However, if one wishes to investigate the mechanisms of recovery, it is important to document the induced changes as carefully and in as detailed a fashion as possible. For example, although patients may perform well on ADL tasks, they may still exhibit reduced skillfulness of an affected hand, despite regaining the ability to solve simple spatial motor problems (Platz et al, 1994). Although it is essential to know whether a patient becomes independent, it is also of importance to know, for example, what effect the motor and sensory experience of physiotherapy has on the motor system. These are two different questions, the latter being concerned with the relationship between changes in the nervous system and consequent functional recovery. To begin to understand mechanisms of recovery and potentially to be able to manipulate these mechanisms, one must look beyond using ADL scores as an assessment. This is an important lesson in assessing any form of rehabilitative strategy if we are to avoid discarding potentially useful treatments as a result of selecting poor or inappropriate outcome measures.

## Plasticity in the Normal Brain

When considering mechanisms of recovery after focal brain injury, the term 'plasticity' is often used. Over 50 years ago, Hebb postulated that increments in synaptic efficacy occur during learning, when firing of one neuron repeatedly produces firing in another neuron to which it is connected (Hebb, 1947, 1949). This expresses the notion that a change in behaviour (i.e. learning) is associated with a change of function at the level of the synapse. In a more general framework, a definition of plasticity might specify a change in structure over time with a consequent change in function (Kolb, 1995), and the cortex – with its myriad synaptic connections – is the ideal site for this plasticity to take place (Sanes and Donoghue, 2000). Using this loose definition of plasticity, we can see that changes at the cortical level can occur in a number of ways. Firstly, it has been repeatedly demonstrated that enriched environments and motor learning in adult animals are associated with morphological changes in the cortex, suggesting increases in the number of synaptic connections. These changes include growth of dendrites, increases in dendritic spines and synaptogenesis (Bury et al, 2000; Ivanco and Greenough, 2000). Secondly, echoing the sentiments of Hebb, long-term potentiation (LTP) and long-term depression (LTD) have long been known about as mechanisms of changing synaptic efficacy in the context of learning studies, particularly in the hippocampus (Collingridge and Bliss, 1995).

More recently there has been evidence that these processes can occur in the neocortex if certain conditions, such as a concurrent ascending input, are in place (Hess et al, 1996), and that motor skill learning is accompanied by changes in the strength of connections within primary motor cortex in animal models (Rioult-Pedotti et al, 1998). Lastly, the influence of one cortical neuron on another can be altered by factors other than external environment or practice. Jacobs and Donoghue (1991) performed an experiment in which bicuculline (a GABA antagonist) was applied to the forelimb area of rat motor cortex. Stimulation of the adjacent cortex (normally representing the vibrissa) then leads to forelimb movements. This suggests that cortical maps are maintained at least in part by GABA, and can be altered by pharmacological manipulation.

In studying the human brain there are clearly greater limitations, and very different techniques are needed to study alterations in cortical function and neural networks. Studies using transcranial magnetic stimulation (TMS) have demonstrated changes in cortical function in response to sensory input (Hamdy et al, 1998), motor imagery (Hashimoto and Rothwell, 1999), and motor practice (Pascual-Leone et al, 2000), and functional imaging has been used to demonstrate changes in the organization of neural networks during motor learning (Karni et al, 1995; Toni et al, 1998).

Up to now we have been discussing the potential for plastic change in the normal brain, but it is important to consider whether plasticity also occurs in the damaged brain, and whether this process in any way contributes to functional recovery.

## Plasticity in the Lesioned Brain

A key message that has emerged over the last few years is that the lesioned brain and the normal brain are different when it comes to the potential for plastic change. There is much evidence now to support the idea that the lesioned brain has an increased capacity for plastic change. Developmental proteins not normally expressed in the adult brain re-emerge in the hours and days following focal brain injury. These proteins are involved in changes in the extracellular matrix, structure of glial support cells, neuronal growth, apoptosis, angiogenesis and cellular differentiation (Cramer and Chopp, 2000). Recent work has also demonstrated that following ischaemic damage in adult rats, new progenitor neurons migrate from the subventricular zone and dentate gyrus to the site of damage. Here, these new cells express morphological characteristics of the recently damaged cells (Arvidsson et al, 2002). Structural changes have also been observed, with evidence of neurogenesis (Gould et al, 1999), increased dendritic branching (Jones and Schallert, 1992) and synaptogenesis (Jones et al, 1996). The correlation between some of these changes and behavioural recovery becomes clearer when considering that the magnitude and temporal course of cellular events often parallel this recovery (Cramer and Chopp, 2000). It is also interesting to consider the spatial distribution of such changes, with synaptogenesis (Stroemer et al, 1998) and axonal outgrowth (Kawamata et al, 1997) seen in perilesional tissue in rats, and evidence of dendritic branching in homotopic cortex in the non-lesioned hemisphere (Kozlowski et al, 1996). The changes in cortical structure and function that might mediate recovery may therefore occur at sites distant from the lesion.

The idea that intact areas of the brain become functionally and metabolically inactive because they are disconnected from the site of focal lesions (a phenomenon known as *diaschisis*), and that this might have an impact on the clinical presentation but also on recovery, was first discussed at the beginning of the last century by Von

Monakow in 1914. In a human PET study, survival of the metabolically active cortex surrounding an infarct correlated with neurological recovery in acute stroke patients (Furlan et al, 1996), although the evidence that reversal of diaschisis (rather than recovery of stunned cells in the ischaemic penumbra) contributes to functional recovery is conflicting. Resolution of ipsilateral thalamocortical diaschisis seems to correlate with improvements in cognition and neglect (Baron et al, 1992), but does not seem clearly related to motor outcome; and reversal of crossed cerebellar diaschisis is not related to recovery of motor function (Infeld et al, 1995). Bowler et al (1995) performed SPECT scans in 50 unselected patients with cerebral infarcts at the time of infarct and 3 months later. They could not demonstrate that diaschisis independently added to the clinical deficit after stroke, and they found no correlation between recovery and reduction in diaschisis. However, other forms of metabolic change distant from the site of the lesion have also been observed in animal models. Widespread areas of hyperexcitability in cortex, distinct from the areas of metabolic depression, have been observed in several studies, both ipsilateral and contralateral to the lesion (Witte and Stoll, 1997). In animal models, the extent and time course of recovery of these areas of hyperexcitability do not correlate with the changes in metabolic diaschisis, so they are presumably distinct processes. It has been proposed that it is these areas of hyperexcitability that develop in the first 5 days and partially reverse over months, that may be the substrate for use-dependent plasticity (Witte, 1998). Hagemann et al (1998) demonstrated that the induction of long-term potentiation (LTP) is facilitated in similar hyperexcitable cortical areas in the surround of focal cortical infarcts in rats in vitro, associated with and probably mediated by reduced GABAergic inhibition and increased NMDA receptor-mediated glutamate response. In this hyperexcitable cortex, inputs from neighbouring cortical neurons may become more efficacious, shifting the cortical map. However, taking advantage of this hyperexcitable state and the induction of LTP is likely to require task-related activation by training. That potential mechanism of recovery is not established, but the link is tantalizing.

In human studies, using different techniques, there is also evidence of changes in the organization of cortical networks following focal brain lesions. Enlargement of cortical motor maps demonstrated with TMS correlates with functional improvement in stroke patients (Traversa et al, 1997), and changes in activation maps of recovered patients post-stroke have been demonstrated in both motor (Weiller et al, 1993; Cramer et al, 1997) and language studies (Warburton et al, 1999). However, as yet there is no direct evidence to suggest that the lesioned human brain has an increased capacity for plastic change compared to the unlesioned brain. Furthermore, many of the animal models mentioned are models of cortical damage, and it is not clear that these data are relevant to subcortical stroke. However, the data that are available from animal models encourage us to speculate that we may be able to take advantage of changes in the human lesioned brain to promote functional recovery.

## Promoting Functional Recovery after Stroke

Given that the brain has the capacity for plastic change, and that this seems to increase in the lesioned brain as a consequence of expression of trophic factors and other changes, how might we take advantage of such changes to influence outcome? A number of studies have demonstrated that these changes are dependent not only on the lesion, but on experiential demand (Schallert et al, 2000). For example, in rats subjected to unilateral sensorimotor cortex damage, restraining of the impaired forelimb leads to reduced dendritic arborization in surrounding cortical tissue. This is not seen if the impaired limb continues to be used (Jones and Schallert, 1992).

Animal studies have been supportive of the idea of task-specific training effects in cortically injured subjects, and have begun to shed light on the underlying mechanisms. Nudo et al (1996), in an important study, trained squirrel monkeys in the execution of a complex motor task using a hand. Focal infarcts of a small portion of the hand representation in cortex were induced and 5 days later intensive retraining identical to that previously applied was undertaken. This continued until pre-infarct levels of performance were attained. Using intracortical microstimulation techniques, they found that spared hand areas had either been preserved or had expanded into regions previously occupied by elbow and shoulder representations. Animals in whom retraining had not been attempted and in whom recovery had been less marked had lost remaining hand representation in the cortex. Rehabilitative training would therefore seem to have had an effect on reorganization of intact cortex, as measured by changes in cortical maps, with a consequent beneficial effect on motor recovery. Exposure of animals to an enriched environment enhances dendritic growth and synapse formation (Schallert et al, 2000), and has also been demonstrated to enhance recovery after brain injury (Ohlsson and Johansson, 1995). This effect is likely to be related to experience and consequent cognitive processing, as physical exercise on its own does not produce such significant results on post-injury motor recovery (Gentile et al, 1987).

Parallels exist in human studies, as has already been mentioned. In particular, improvements in motor performance in the chronic setting have been demonstrated with constraint-induced therapy (CIT), based on overcoming learned non-use of the affected limb (Taub et al, 1993), and have been accompanied by increases in cortical representation of the affected limb (Liepert et al, 2000). Other theoretically derived techniques, such as bilateral arm training, are similarly under investigation (Whitall et al, 2000). Underpinning all these techniques is the concept of activity-driven change, the notion that by increasing the activity of neurons in strategically located cortical regions, structural change will ensue, resulting in improvement of function. A striking example is that of an increase in pinch grip strength induced by 2 hours of median nerve stimulation in hemiparetic patients (Conforto et al, 2002). This notion is useful yet likely to be oversimplified. Many aspects of language and motor function in the normal brain are still under active investigation. Motor learning, for example, is the product of complex dynamic interactions between cortical and subcortical structures, which is likely to be optimized by certain conditions and learning techniques (Hikosaka et al, 2002). Until we have an empirical understanding of these optimal parameters in both health and disease, our attempts to promote functional recovery will not have the well grounded theoretical basis that is required for progress.

A critical issue concerns the timing of interventions. The evidence presented seems to suggest that many of the changes that take place after stroke, the very changes that we may need to take advantage of to promote functional change, occur early after the lesion. Therefore it would seem likely that, to take full advantage of these changes, intervention must occur relatively soon after stroke. However, there has been a reluctance to use many interventions (such as forced therapy) in the acute setting because of alternate evidence that such an approach may lead to exacerbation of cortical damage (Kozlowski et al, 1996). This overuse-dependent exaggeration of injury can be blocked by administering MK-801 (an NMDA antagonist), suggesting that glutaminergic mechanisms are involved. The question of timing of an intervention may therefore be critical, because there are definite changes in the molecular and cellular environment at a certain time point after injury. For example, it has been hypothesized that during early development new synapses with high NMDA:AMPA receptor ratios are formed. This ratio rapidly becomes similar to that seen in adults. In any period where new synapses are forming – such as early development, new learning, or after focal brain damage (Stroemer et al, 1998) – use-dependent plasticity is likely to occur in the new synapses with high NMDA: AMPA receptor ratios, which may explain why NMDA antagonists, although thought to be protective in acute ischaemia, may slow or prevent plastic changes occurring in perilesional tissue, with subsequent impairment of functional recovery (Barth et al, 1990). Understanding of these processes is crucial if we are to use interventions correctly.

It is worth considering that the capacity for plastic change in any brain may be finite, particularly with ageing. Functional imaging studies have examined for differences in recruitment of brain regions during both motor (Mattay et al, 2002) and cognitive tasks (D'Esposito et al, 1999), and many of these studies have found greater activations in a number of regions in older subjects when compared with younger subjects. However, this may only be the case for those older subjects whose level of performance is comparable to that in the younger subjects (Mattay et al, 2002). It has been suggested that interruption of the normal neural networks subserving cognitive performance by age-related neurodegenerative and neurochemical changes underlies decline in function (Wenk et al, 1989; Volkow et al, 1998); but that compensatory processes in cortical and subcortical function allow maintenance of performance level in some people. We also know that after injury-induced reorganization of the brain, the capacity for subsequent adaptive change is reduced (Kolb et al, 1998a). It is possible that the adaptive changes that have been observed in older brains and injured brains may in turn limit the capacity for further reorganization after injury. This clearly has implications for what we can expect from therapeutic techniques designed to promote cerebral reorganization after stroke in older subjects. A greater understanding of age-related changes in the functional reorganization of the brain will be crucial in unravelling the relationship between normal ageing and pathological process.

# Pharmacological Manipulation of Recovery after Stroke

## Animal models

There has been long-standing interest in whether the processes collectively described as neuronal or synaptic plasticity can be influenced by pharmacological manipulation. As early as 1942, investigators concluded that the cholinergic drugs, strychnine and thiamine, could enhance the rate and degree of recovery from motor cortex damage in monkeys (Ward and Kennard, 1942). However, by the 1950s it was felt that pharmacological stimulation of the reticular activating system was the key to facilitating recovery. Amphetamine was first used by Maling and Acheson (1946), who demonstrated that this drug transiently restored righting reflexes in low decerebrate cats, and subsequently Meyer et al, (1963) temporarily restored the placing reflex in decorticate cats by the administration of amphetamine, 1 year after they had originally undergone surgery. Faugier-Grimaud et al (1978) also demonstrated that a deficit could be temporarily reinduced after recovery had taken place. They performed either unilateral or bilateral parietal lesions in Java monkeys, inducing deficits in visually guided reaching tasks, after which spontaneous recovery took 2 weeks. One year after surgery the monkeys were given a small dose of the general anaesthetic, ketamine, which resulted in an immediate but temporary return of the deficit, with the deficit being unilateral or bilateral depending on the number of lesions performed 1 year previously.

Feeney and co-workers (1982) revisited amphetamine as a possible neuromodulator of functional recovery. A series of experiments were carried out on rats that had undergone suction ablation of the sensorimotor cortex. Amphetamine given after ablation and rehabilitative practice both appeared to speed up recovery significantly, but crucially rehabilitative practice contributed to this effect only in the context of amphetamine administration, and vice versa. Haloperidol given with amphetamine blocked the effect, and given alone retarded recovery, suggesting a role for dopamine (DA) neurotransmission. Further observations implicated the cerebellum in this effect. Firstly, both amphetamine and haloperidol worsen beam walking recovery in rats with cerebellar injury (Boyeson and Feeney, 1991), and secondly microinfusions of noradrenaline (NA) into the cerebellum (contralateral but not ipsilateral to the site of a cortical injury) mimic the systemic effects of drugs on beam walking recovery in rats (Boyeson and Krobert, 1992).

Although the effect of haloperidol in Feeney's initial experiments suggested that the effect was mediated by DA, further evidence implicates NA. Lesions to the contralateral but not ipsilateral dorsal noradrenergic bundle (projecting from the locus coeruleus to the cerebral cortex), impair motor recovery after subsequent cortical lesion (Goldstein and Bullman, 1997). Alpha-2 antagonists (increasing noradrenergic effect) such as yohimbine and idazoxan have also been found to facilitate motor recovery in a single dose (Sutton and Feeney, 1992). Conversely, drugs that decrease NA release in the central nervous system, or block post-synaptic effects (i.e. alpha-1 antagonists/alpha-2 agonists), are likely to be harmful to recovery in the above model, and in fact clonidine (alpha-2 agonist) (Goldstein and Davis, 1990) impairs beam walking recovery, in the same way as haloperidol. In an echo of the work done by Faugier-Grimaud et al in 1978, it was noted that these drugs not only impair recovery, but if given to a rat that has made a spontaneous recovery, will reinstate the deficit temporarily, to a degree proportional to the original deficit. This effect has been seen with several drugs (clonidine, prazosin, phenoxybenzamine) and across species (Feeney, 1997).

Speculation as to the mechanism of action of these effects is fascinating. Noradrenergic-induced changes in local metabolism or enhancement of LTP may allow motor experience to induce permanent changes. We have already discussed the evidence pointing towards how this may occur in relation to LTP (Hagemann et al, 1998). It is also fascinating to note that the effects of neurotransmitters (and drugs that affect these neurotransmitters) on LTP induction correlate strongly with their effects on recovery of function after sensorimotor cortex injury in animals (Goldstein, 1990). More recently Stroemer and co-workers (1998) induced unilateral cortical ischaemia in a group of rats, and then treated one group with amphetamine and one with saline. Levels of GAP-43 and synaptophysin, as markers of neurite growth and synaptogenesis, respectively, were measured in peri-infarct tissue at different intervals after the lesion was induced. Behavioural recovery was measured at the same time intervals. Levels of GAP-43 and synaptophysin were found to be significantly elevated and the degree of elevation correlated with behavioural recovery in a temporal fashion. It is tempting therefore to suggest that the increase in expression of these proteins promotes structural change (as the possible substrate of recovery) directly, but it is known that these proteins are associated also with release of NA and DA (Dekker et al, 1989), and possibly with LTP (Iwata et al, 1997), both of which may be important factors themselves in functional recovery.

The fact that the recovery of function is so susceptible to reversal by pharmacological agents (e.g. ketamine, prazosin, clonidine), suggests that changes are not purely anatomical and that a change in the neurochemical balance of interacting systems has been effected. Both Luria (1963) and Meyer (1972) have suggested that lesions in these animal models cause a suppression of retrieval of motor engrams, which have been formed in the brain as a result of previous learning and experience. Perhaps these motor engrams are not destroyed by cortical lesions but become inaccessible, and noradrenergic enhancement allows them to be accessed once more. This is of course speculation, but it is a hypothesis that addresses the problem of assuming that localized cortical changes can substitute for profound disturbances in distributed networks. Restoration of dynamic interactions between the nodes of these networks is likely to be crucial in regaining meaningful recovery. Indirect evidence to support this comes not only from systems neuroscience, but also from cellular and molecular studies. New neuronal cells migrating to the site of damage following middle cerebral artery occlusion in rats express the morphological characteristics of neurons that form part of the basal ganglia–cortical loops, so important in motor control (Arvidsson et al, 2002).

There is also evidence that modulation of other neurotransmitter systems can have similar effects. Dopamine has already been mentioned in relation to Feeney's work with haloperidol. Apomorphine reduces the severity of experimentally induced neglect from prefrontal injury, and spiroperidol reinstates this neglect (Feeney, 1997). GABA infused intracortically impairs beam walking recovery in rats (Brailowsky et al, 1986), and diazepam impairs recovery of sensory asymmetry caused by unilateral damage to the anteromedial cortex in rats (Schallert et al, 1986). The acetylcholine antagonist scopolamine interferes with recovery after motor cortex infarction in rats (De Ryck et al, 1990), and in monkeys, cholinergic drugs increase the rate of recovery in animals with motor cortex lesions (Watson and Kennard, 1945). The NMDA antagonist MK-801, has been found to be detrimental if given during the recovery period in rats (Barth et al, 1990), which is in contrast to its proposed neuroprotective effect if given immediately after an infarct.

More recently, a greater understanding of the molecular and cellular events occurring post injury has led to attempts to manipulate them for the purposes of promoting functional recovery. Candidate compounds include osteogenic protein-1 (Ren et al, 2000), brain-derived neurotrophic factor (Rossi et al, 1999), fibroblast growth factor-2 (Kawamata et al, 1997) and stem cell treatment (Kolb et al, 1998b).

In summary, experiments in animals point most strongly towards the influence of neurotransmitter systems on functional recovery after focal brain injury. The effect is dose dependent, and the timing of administration is crucial, with the effect being dependent on close temporal linkage to behavioural experience.

## Human studies

What of attempts to translate these findings into promotion of functional recovery in humans? Much of the early work in this field has been done by Alexander Luria and colleagues in soldiers with head injuries sustained during the second world war (Luria, 1963; Luria et al, 1963). They proposed two types of functional disturbance as a result of focal brain lesions, i.e. cell death and functional inhibition of intact neurons. They suggested that patients in whom the latter predominated might benefit from 'removal of the diaschisis, restoration of synaptic conduction or to use another term, de-blocking' (Luria et al, 1963). It was proposed that this could be achieved by the combination of two approaches. Firstly the administration of a pharmacological agent 'capable of removing inhibition, modifying mediator metabolism, and restoring disturbed synaptic conduction' (Luria et al, 1963), and secondly by methods of training which promote 'de-blocking', the essence of which is 'that by means of various methods the level of excitability in certain functional systems is raised and the corresponding functions are "de-inhibited"' (Luria et al, 1963). The main de-blocking agents used by these investigators were anticholinesterases. In one such experiment, neostigmine was administered to a patient with a non-penetrating wound of the premotor area. Rhythmic tapping movements were recorded before and after neostigmine was given, and improvements of 'dynamic co-ordination' were noted after the drug, when none had been obtained with repeated training attempts prior to this experiment (Luria, 1963). Luria also made claims that the rate of recovery from aphasia could be increased (as long as the lesion was not in what he described as the 'primary speech areas') using galantamine (a specific, competitive and reversible acetylcholinesterase inhibitor now under investigation for the treatment of dementia) (Luria, 1963).

It is surprising that, despite this large body of work, further studies of pharmacological enhancement of recovery were not pursued further until nearly 40 years after Luria's original work was published. The first trial of noradrenergic enhancement coupled with physical therapy in human subjects was published in 1988 (Crisostomo et al, 1988). In this experiment patients who had suffered from hemiplegic stroke were randomized to receive 10 mg amphetamine or placebo, 45 minutes prior to physiotherapy. Follow-up assessment 24 hours after treatment indicated a 40% improvement from baseline scores compared with placebo. The small numbers of patients in this study (eight in total), make interpretation difficult, as the authors stated. A subsequent failure to replicate these findings by Borucki et al (1992) was attributed to different experimental design, in particular a failure to schedule physiotherapy immediately after amphetamine treatment. Perhaps also significant, in view of the possible therapeutic window, was that treatment was not started until over a month after the stroke. More recent studies with d-amphetamine have had conflicting results (Walker-Batson et al, 1995; Sonde et al, 2001), but positive results have been published for daily doses of L-dopa (100 mg) used in conjunction with physiotherapy (Scheidtmann et al, 2001). Studies have initially focused on motor recovery, most likely because of obvious parallels with animal studies, but similar studies looking at recovery in aphasia post stroke have been performed (Walker-Batson et al, 2001).

Following on from the idea that exogenously administered drugs may alter the balance of extracellular concentrations of various neurotransmitters, and that this might in turn have an effect on functional outcome following focal brain injury via an as yet undetermined mechanism, Goldstein et al (1990) performed a retrospective analysis of the effect of drugs (predicted from animal models to have a deleterious effect on motor outcome following focal brain injury) on outcome in stroke patients. Patients receiving phenytoin, benzodiazepines or alpha-adrenergic antihypertensive agents at the time of stroke or shortly afterwards had poorer outcomes than the controls who did not receive any of these drugs. This was found to be the case for a number of outcome measures, covering both ADLs and specific motor function, and 30-day recovery rates. These findings were replicated by the Acute Stroke Study Investigators

(Goldstein, 1995), using a group of patients who were themselves the control group in a prospective acute interventional trial. Forty percent of these patients received one or a combination of drugs predicted to impair recovery, and were found to have poorer recovery as assessed by a variety of measures. Similar findings have been published relating to the adverse effects of certain antihypertensive agents (Porch and Feeney, 1986). These analyses were retrospective and could not exclude the possibility that patients were given these drugs for medical reasons that themselves would predict poorer outcome, but this area of research clearly warrants further investigation.

Evidence therefore exists that certain drugs influence behavioural recovery in humans following focal brain injury. This has implications in as much as it suggests that more could be done to enhance recovery in these patients, and also that certain drugs are probably best avoided in these circumstances.

## Summary

Until recently it has been on the basis of intuition rather than evidence that physicians have recommended post-acute therapy for stroke patients. Evidence now exists that stroke units work, and that specific retraining techniques have measurable benefits. A wealth of evidence has been produced from work in animal models that the lesioned brain changes at a molecular, cellular and systems level, in a way that promotes experientially driven changes in synaptic structure and function. There is clearly a bias towards motor studies in animal models, but the principle of a post-lesional plastic brain applies to any cortical function. Many questions remain unanswered, including whether the older human brain also has this capacity for plastic change, and the challenge is now to advance our understanding of the science of recovery after brain damage in humans, and crucially how we can use this information to promote recovery.

## References

Arvidsson A, Collin T, Kirik D, Kokaia Z, Lindvall O (2002) Neuronal replacement from endogenous precursors in the adult brain after stroke. *Nature Medicine* **8**: 963–70.

Baron J-C, Levasseur M, Mazoyer B et al (1992) Thalamocortical diaschisis: positron emission tomography in humans. *Journal of Neurology Neurosurgery and Psychiatry* **55**: 935–42.

Barth TM, Grant ML, Schallert T (1990) Effects of MK-801 on recovery from sensorimotor cortex lesions. *Stroke* **21**: 153–7.

Bonita R, Solomon N, Broad JB (1997) Prevalence of stroke and stroke-related disability: estimates from The Auckland Stroke Study. *Stroke* **28**: 1898–902.

Borucki SJ, Landberg J, Redinng M (1992) The effect of dextroamphetamine on motor recovery after stroke. *Neurology* **42**: (Suppl 3): 329.

Bowler JV, Wade JP, Jones BE et al (1995) Contribution of diaschisis to the clinical deficit in human cerebral infarction. *Stroke* **26**: 1000–6.

Boyeson MG, Feeney DM (1991) Adverse effects of catacholaminergic agonists and antagonists on recovery of locomotor ability following unilateral cerebellar ablations. *Restorative Neurology and Neuroscience* **3**: 227–33.

Boyeson MG, Krobert KA (1992) Cerebellar norepinephrine infusions facilitate recovery after sensorimotor cortex injury. *Brain Research Bulletin* **29**: 435–9.

Brailowsky S, Knight RT, Blood K, Scabini D (1986) gamma-Aminobutyric acid-induced potentiation of cortical hemiplegia. *Brain Research* **362**: 322–30.

Brown MM (2002) Brain attack: a new approach to stroke. *Clinical Medicine* **2**: 60–5.

Bury SD, Eichhorn AC, Kotzer CM, Jones TA (2000) Reactive astrocytic responses to denervation in the motor cortex of adult rats are sensitive to manipulations of behavioral experience. *Neuropharmacology* **39**: 743–55.

Collingridge GL, Bliss TV (1995) Memories of NMDA receptors and LTP. *Trends in Neurosciences* **18**: 54–6.

Conforto AB, Kaelin-Lang A, Cohen LG (2002) Increase in hand muscle strength of stroke patients after somatosensory stimulation. *Annals of Neurology* **51**: 122–5.

Cramer SC, Nelles G, Benson RR et al (1997) A functional MRI study of subjects recovered from hemiparetic stroke. *Stroke* **28**: 2518–27.

Cramer SC, Chopp M (2000). Recovery recapitulates ontogeny. *Trends in Neurosciences* **23**: 265–71.

Crisostomo EA, Duncan PW, Propst M, Dawson DV, Davis JN (1988) Evidence that amphetamine with physical therapy promotes recovery of motor function in stroke patients. *Annals of Neurology* **23**: 94–7.

Dekker LV, De Graan PN, Oestreicher AB, Versteeg DH, Gispen WH (1989) Inhibition of noradrenaline release by antibodies to B-50 (GAP-43). *Nature* **342**: 74–6.

De Ryck M, Duytschaever H, Pauwels PJ, Janssen PA (1990) Ionic channels, cholinergic mechanisms, and recovery of sensorimotor function after neocortical infarcts in rats. *Stroke* **21**: 158–63.

D'Esposito M, Zarahn E, Aguirre GK, Rypma B (1999) The effect of normal aging on the coupling of neural activity to the bold hemodynamic response. *Neuroimage* **10**: 6–14.

Faugier-Grimaud S, Frenois C, Stein DG (1978) Effects of posterior parietal lesions on visually guided behaviour in monkeys. *Neuropsychologia* **16**: 151–68.

Feeney DM (1997) From laboratory to clinic: noradrenergic enhancement of physical therapy for stroke or trauma patients. *Advances in Neurology* **73**: 383–94.

Feeney DM, Gonzalez A, Law WA (1982) Amphetamine, haloperidol, and experience interact to affect rate of recovery after motor cortex injury. *Science* **217**: 855–7.

Furlan M, Marchal G, Viader F, Derlon JM, Baron JC (1996) Spontaneous neurological recovery after stroke and the fate of the ischaemic penumbra. *Annals of Neurology* **40**: 216–26.

Gentile AM, Beheshti Z, Held JM (1987) Enrichment versus exercise effects on motor impairments following cortical removals in rats. *Behavioural and Neural Biology* **47**: 321–32.

Goldstein LB (1990) Pharmacology of recovery after stroke. *Stroke* **21**: 139–42.

Goldstein LB (1995) Common drugs may influence motor recovery after stroke. The Sygen In Acute Stroke Study Investigators. *Neurology* **45**: 865–71.

Goldstein LB, Bullman S (1997) Effects of dorsal noradrenergic bundle lesions on recovery after sensorimotor cortex injury. *Pharmacology, Biochemistry and Behavior* **58**: 1151–7.

Goldstein LB, Davis JN (1990) Clonidine impairs recovery of beam-walking after a sensorimotor cortex lesion in the rat. *Brain Research* **508**: 305–9.

Goldstein LB, Matchar DB, Morgenlander JC, Davis JN (1990) The influence of drugs on the recovery of sensorimotor function after stroke. *Journal of Neurologic Rehabilitation* **4**: 137–44.

Gould E, Reeves AJ, Graziano MS, Gross CG (1999) Neurogenesis in the neocortex of adult primates. *Science* **286**: 548–52.

Hagemann G, Redecker C, Neumann-Haefelin T, Freund HJ, Witte OW (1998) Increased long-term potentiation in the surround of experimentally induced focal cortical infarction. *Annals of Neurology* **44**: 255–8.

Hamdy S, Rothwell JC, Aziz Q, Singh KD, Thompson DG (1998) Long-term reorganization of human motor cortex driven by short-term sensory stimulation. *Nature Neuroscience* **1**: 64–8.

Hashimoto R, Rothwell JC (1999) Dynamic changes in corticospinal excitability during motor imagery. *Experimental Brain Research* **125**: 75–81.

Hebb DO (1947) The effects of early experience on problem solving at maturity. *American Psychologist* **2**: 737–45.

Hebb DO (1949) *The Organisation of Behaviour: A Neuropsychological Theory.* Wiley, New York.

Hess G, Aizenman CD, Donoghue JP (1996) Conditions for the induction of long-term potentiation in layer II/III horizontal connections of the rat motor cortex. *Journal of Neurophysiology* **75**: 1765–78.

Hesse SA, Jahnke MT, Bertelt CM, Schreiner C, Lucke D, Mauritz KH (1994) Gait outcome in ambulatory hemiparetic patients after a 4-week comprehensive rehabilitation program and prognostic factors. *Stroke* **25**: 1999–2004.

Hesse S, Malezic M, Schaffrin A, Mauritz KH (1995) Restoration of gait by combined treadmill training and multichannel electrical stimulation in non-ambulatory hemiparetic patients. *Scandanavian Journal of Rehabilitation Medicine* **27**: 199–204.

Hikosaka O, Nakamura K, Sakai K, Nakahara H (2002) Central mechanisms of motor skill learning. *Current Opinion in Neurobiology* **12**: 217–22.

Infeld B, Davis SM, Lichtenstein M, Mitchell PJ, Hopper JL (1995) Crossed cerebellar diaschisis and brain recovery after stroke. *Stroke* **26**: 90–5.

Ivanco TL, Greenough WT (2000) Physiological consequences of morphologically detectable synaptic plasticity: potential uses for examining recovery following damage. *Neuropharmacology* **39**: 765–76.

Iwata SI, Hewlett GH, Ferrell ST, Kantor L, Gnegy ME (1997) Enhanced dopamine release and phosphorylation of synaptophysin I and neuromodulin in striatal synaptosomes after repeated amphetamine. *Journal of Pharmacology and Experimental Therapeutics* **283**: 1445–52.

Jacobs KM, Donoghue JP (1991) Reshaping the cortical motor map by unmasking latent intracortical connections. *Science* **251**: 944–7.

Jones TA, Schallert T (1992) Overgrowth and pruning of dendrites in adult rats recovering from neocortical damage. *Brain Research* **581**: 156–60.

Jones TA, Kleim JA, Greenough WT (1996) Synaptogenesis and dendritic growth in the cortex opposite unilateral sensorimotor cortex damage in adult rats: a quantitative electron microscopic examination. *Brain Research* **733**: 142–8.

Karni A, Meyer G, Jezzard P, Adams MM, Turner R, Ungerleider LG (1995) Functional MRI evidence for adult motor cortex plasticity during motor skill learning. *Nature* **377**: 155–8.

Kawamata T, Dietrich WD, Schallert T et al (1997) Intracisternal basic fibroblast growth factor enhances functional recovery and up-regulates the expression of a molecular marker of neuronal sprouting following focal cerebral infarction. *Proceedings of the National Academy of Science USA* **94**: 8179–84.

Kolb B (1995) *Brain Plasticity and Behaviour*, 1–194. Lawrence Erlbaum, Mahwah, NJ.

Kolb B, Forgie M, Gibb R, Gorny G, Rowntree S (1998a) Age, experience and the changing brain. *Neuroscience and Biobehavioural Reviews* **22**: 143–159.

Kolb B, Gibb R, Biernaskie J, Dyck RH, Whishaw IQ (1998b) Regeneration of olfactory bulb or frontal cortex in infant and adult rats. *Abstracts Society for Neuroscience* **24**: 518.

Kozlowski DA, James DC, Schallert T (1996) Use-dependent exaggeration of neuronal injury after unilateral sensorimotor cortex lesions. *Journal of Neuroscience* **16**: 4776–86.

Kwakkel G, Wagenaar RC, Koelman TW, Lankhorst GJ, Koetsier JC (1997) Effects of intensity of rehabilitation after stroke. A research synthesis. *Stroke* **28**: 1550–6.

Kwakkel G, Wagenaar RC, Twisk JW, Lankhorst GJ, Koetsier JC (1999) Intensity of leg and arm training after primary middle-cerebral-artery stroke: a randomised trial. *Lancet* **354**: 191–6.

Langhorne P, Wagenaar R, Partridge C (1996) Physiotherapy after stroke: more is better? *Physiotherapy Research International* **1**: 75–88.

Lees KR (2000) Thrombolysis. In: Brown MM ed. Stroke. *British Medical Bulletin* **56**: 389–400.

Liepert J, Graef S, Uhde I, Leidner O, Weiller C (2000) Training-induced changes of motor cortex representations in stroke patients. *Acta Neurologica Scandanavica* **101**: 321–6.

Luria AR (1963) Restoration of Function after Brain Injury. Pergamon Press, Oxford.

Luria AR, Naydin VL, Tsvetkova LS, Vinarskaya EN (1963) Restoration of higher cortical function following local brain damage. In: Vinken PJ, Bruyn GW, eds. *Handbook of Clinical Neurology*, Vol 3, 368–433. North Holland Publishing Company, Amsterdam.

Maling HM, Acheson GH (1946) Righting and other postural activity in low decerebrate and in spinal cats after d-amphetamime. *Journal of Neurophysiology* **9**: 379–86.

Mattay VS, Fera F, Tessitore A et al (2002) Neurophysiological correlates of age-related changes in human motor function. *Neurology* **58**: 630–5.

Meyer DR (1972) Access to engrams. *American Psychologist* **27**: 124–33.

Meyer PM, Horel JA, Meyer DR (1963) Effects of d-amphetamine upon placing responses in neodecorticate cats. *Journal of Comparative and Physiological Psychology* **56**: 402–4.

Nudo RJ, Wise BM, SiFuentes F, Milliken GW (1996) Neural substrates for the effects of rehabilitative training on motor recovery after ischemic infarct. *Science* **272**: 1791–4.

Ohlsson AL, Johansson BB (1995) Environment influences functional outcome of cerebral infarction in rats. *Stroke* **26**: 644–9.

O'Mahoney PG, Thomson RG, Dobson R, Rodgers H, James OF (1999) The prevalence of stroke and associated disability. *Journal of Public Health Medicine* **21**: 166–71.

Pascual-Leone A, Walsh V, Rothwell J (2000) Transcranial magnetic stimulation in cognitive neuroscience – virtual lesion, chronometry, and functional connectivity. *Current Opinion in Neurobiology* **10**: 232–7.

Platz T, Denzler P, Kaden B, Mauritz KH (1994) Motor learning after recovery from hemiparesis. *Neuropsychologia* **32**: 1209–23.

Porch BE, Feeney DM (1986) The effects of antihypertensive drugs on recovery from aphasia. *Clinical Aphasiology* **16**: 309–14.

Ren J, Kaplan PL, Charette MF, Spellerm H, Finklestein SP (2000) Time window of intracisternal osteogenic protein-1 in enhancing functional recovery after stroke. *Neuropharmacology* **39**: 860–5.

Rioult-Pedotti MS, Friedman D, Hess G, Donoghue JP (1998) Strengthening of horizontal cortical connections following skill learning. *Nature Neuroscience* **1**: 230–4.

Rossi FM, Bozzi Y, Pizzorusso T, Maffei L (1999) Monocular deprivation decreases brain-derived neurotrophic factor immunoreactivity in the rat visual cortex. *Neuroscience* **90**: 363–8.

Sanes JN, Donoghue JP (2000) Plasticity and primary motor cortex. *Annual Review of Neuroscience* **23**: 393–415.

Schallert T, Hernandez TD, Barth TM (1986) Recovery of function after brain damage: severe and chronic disruption by diazepam. *Brain Research* **379**: 104–11.

Schallert T, Leasure JL, Kolb B (2000) Experience-associated structural events, subependymal cellular proliferative activity, and functional recovery after injury to the central nervous system. *Journal of Cerebral Blood Flow and Metabolism* **20**: 1513–28.

Scheidtmann K, Fries W, Muller F, Koenig E (2001) Effect of levodopa in combination with physiotherapy on functional motor recovery after stroke: a prospective, randomised, double-blind study. *Lancet* **358**: 787–90.

Smith MT, Baer GD (1999) Achievement of simple mobility milestones after stroke. *Archives of Physical Medicine and Rehabilitation* **80**: 442–7.

Sonde L, Nordstrom M, Nilsson CG, Lokk J, Viitanen M (2001) A double-blind placebo-controlled study of the effects of amphetamine and physiotherapy after stroke. *Cerebrovascular Disease* **12**: 253–7.

Stroemer RP, Kent TA, Hulsebosch CE (1998) Enhanced neocortical neural sprouting, synaptogenesis, and behavioral recovery with D-amphetamine therapy after neocortical infarction in rats. *Stroke* **29**: 2381–93.

Stroke Unit Trialists Collaboration (1997) How do stroke units improve patient outcomes? A collaborative systematic review of the randomized trials. *Stroke* **28**: 2139–44.

Stroke Unit Trialists' Collaboration (2000) Organised inpatient (stroke unit) care for stroke. *Cochrane Database Systematic Review* (2): CD000197.

Sutton RL, Feeney DM (1992) α-Noradrenergic agonists and antagonists affect recovery and maintainance of beam walking ability after sensorimotor cortex ablation in the rat. *Restorative Neurology and Neuroscience* **4**: 1–11.

Taub E, Miller NE, Novack TA et al (1993) Technique to improve chronic motor deficit after stroke. *Archives of Physical Medicine and Rehabilitation* **74**: 347–54.

Toni I, Krams M, Turner R, Passingham RE (1998) The time course of changes during motor sequence learning: a whole-brain fMRI study. *Neuroimage* **8**: 50–61.

Traversa R, Cicinelli P, Bassi A, Rossini PM, Bernardi G (1997) Mapping of motor cortical reorganization after stroke. A brain stimulation study with focal magnetic pulses. *Stroke* **28**: 110–7.

Twitchell TE (1951) The restoration of motor function following hemiplegia in man. *Brain* **74**: 443–80.

Volkow ND, Gur RC, Wang GJ et al (1998) Association between decline in brain dopamine activity with age and cognitive and motor impairment in healthy individuals. *American Journal of Psychiatry* **155**: 344–9.

Von Monakow C (1914) Diaschisis. Translated by G Harris (1969) In: Pribrom KH, ed. *Brain and Behaviour I: Moods, States and Mind*, 27–62. Penguin, Baltimore.

Walker-Batson D, Smith P, Curtis S, Unwin H, Greenlee R (1995) Amphetamine paired with physical therapy accelerates motor recovery after stroke. Further evidence. *Stroke* **26**: 2254–9.

Walker-Batson D, Curtis S, Natarajan R et al (2001) A double-blind, placebo-controlled study of the use of amphetamine in the treatment of aphasia. *Stroke* **32**: 2093–8.

Warburton E, Price CJ, Swinburn K, Wise RJ (1999) Mechanisms of recovery from aphasia: evidence from positron emission tomography studies. *Journal of Neurology Neurosurgery and Psychiatry* **66**: 155–61.

Ward AA Jr, Kennard MA (1942) Effect of cholinergic drugs on recovery of function following lesions of the central nervous system. *Yale Journal of Biology and Medicine* **15**: 189–228.

Watson CW, Kennard MA (1945) The effect of anticonvulsant drugs on recovery of function following cerebral cortical lesions. *Journal of Neurophysiology* **8**: 221–31.

Weiller C, Ramsay SC, Wise RJS, Friston KJ, Frackowiak RSJ (1993) Individual patterns of functional reorganisation in the human cerebral cortex after capsular infarction. *Annals of Neurology* **33**: 181–9.

Wenk GL, Pierce DJ, Struble RG, Price DL, Cork LC (1989). Age-related changes in multiple neurotransmitter systems in the monkey brain. *Neurobiology of Aging* **10**: 11–19.

Whitall J, McCombe Waller S, Silver KH, Macko RF (2000) Repetitive bilateral arm training with rhythmic auditory cueing improves motor function in chronic hemiparetic stroke. *Stroke* **31**: 2390–5.

Witte OW, Stoll G (1997) Delayed and remote effects of focal cortical infarctions: secondary damage and reactive plasticity. *Advances in Neurology* **73**: 207–27.

Witte OW (1998) Lesion-induced plasticity as a potential mechanism for recovery and rehabilitative training. *Current Opinion in Neurology* **11**: 655–62.

# 2

# An Interdisciplinary Team Approach to Acute Stroke Rehabilitation

*Sarah Guy, Linsey Clarke, Helena Bryant, Gail Robinson, Ella Segaran, Nick Losseff and Trudy Stewart*

## Introduction

There is significant evidence that organized stroke units are effective in improving outcome. The findings of the Stroke Unit Trialists Collaboration (1997, 2000), based on a meta-analysis, indicate that the management of patients with stroke within a dedicated unit reduces mortality and morbidity with no definite increase in length of stay.

It is not immediately clear why organized stroke services are successful, but several distinct features have been identified in these studies which characterize organized care as opposed to that delivered within a general setting. A stroke unit typically incorporates a multidisciplinary team who have a specific interest in assessment and management of patients following stroke. This team will have a level of expertise with regards to this clinical area and are likely to have access to internal and external training. Within stroke units, guidelines will exist based on agreed, evidence-based protocols, specific to the management of patients who have had stroke.

The team will have ownership of the patient's problems and are likely to advocate an active approach. Communication between the team will be coordinated both by meetings and by sharing a dedicated geographic space. Therefore goals and discharge planning are common to all members. It is these features, which stem from 'organization' of care, that have been suggested to play a fundamental role in the successful outcomes achieved by stroke units.

This chapter aims to outline the role of the interdisciplinary team in the management of stroke patients following one possible model of care. It is not possible to provide a 'recipe' for stroke rehabilitation, as each patient should have a treatment plan based on his or her individual needs. The aim of this chapter is to discuss the practical features of teamworking and patient care in stroke rehabilitation, based on available evidence. The chapter focuses on the assessment and rehabilitation of patients following stroke in the acute inpatient setting (within the first 6 weeks of stroke onset). However, many of the principles discussed will also apply to teams working in other inpatient and community settings.

## The Interdisciplinary Team

A team can be described as a group of individuals working towards a single goal or set of agreed goals (Royal College of Physicians, 2000). Terminology used to describe teams varies depending on their structure. Commonly used terms for team structures in health care are multidisciplinary and interdisciplinary. In recent years there has been a shift from multidisciplinary to interdisciplinary. In a multidisciplinary team, members work independently and patient goals are commonly discipline-specific. Professionals liaise with each other and share information, but tend to work alongside rather than *with* their colleagues. Interdisciplinary team working involves a high level of team communication whereby team members work with each other to set mutual goals for patient care. It is a more integrated way of working with a joint team approach to planning, providing and evaluating patient care (Proctor-Childs et al, 1998).

Interdisciplinary teams evolve from multidisciplinary teams over time and with appropriate leadership. To a large extent they facilitate their own evolution and, although strong leadership is essential, consensus encourages ownership and engagement in the process of development.

The list of professionals included in the interdisciplinary stroke team is not exclusive; many additional professionals are involved in the patients' care including radiographers, phlebotomists and pharmacists, to name but a few. The roles of the most common team members are discussed in detail in relation to stroke rehabilitation. In addition, the patients' families and significant others often play an important role in the rehabilitation process and should be considered as an integral part of the team. By working together, the roles of individual members within the interdisciplinary team will complement each other. Joint working facilitates a more comprehensive assessment, avoiding unnecessary duplication of information and ensuring that patients' rehabilitation is approached in a coordinated manner. This is particularly key in the acute stage when patients may only be able to tolerate short periods of assessment or intervention.

## Nursing staff

The nursing staff are likely to be the first members of the team that the patient and family/significant others make contact with following transfer from the emergency department. The nursing staff play a significant role in coordinating care and offering emotional support to patient and carers (Johnson, 1995). They act as a key link between the patient, the family and the rest of the team. On admission nursing staff orientate the patient and the family to the ward/unit. They assess the patient using the activities of daily living model developed by Roper et al, (1980) to gain a baseline of the patient's initial limitations in activity and participation, in order to identify strengths and needs. The following areas are assessed: neurological status (using the Glasgow Coma Scale), cardiorespiratory function, communication skills, mobility and positioning, nutrition and hydration, elimination, personal self-care skills, pain and sedation needs, infection control issues, presenting mood, behaviour and cognition, and premorbid domestic, work and social level. This comprehensive assessment enables the nursing team to plan their care for each patient; this may include making referrals to other members of the team to address specific needs that have been identified. The nurse also takes primary responsibility, in liaison with the medical team, for assessment and management of bladder and bowel dysfunction, cardiorespiratory function and tissue viability.

## Medical staff

After the nursing staff the next assessment is usually made by the medical staff. Through history, examination and investigation (e.g. blood tests, neuroimaging) they will try and determine the pathophysiology underpinning the clinical presentation, and detail risk factors, comorbidities and complications. The acute phase of stroke treatment should be characterized by careful supportive treatment with optimization of physiological parameters (e.g. blood pressure, hydration, temperature, blood sugar). Appropriate antithrombotic and thrombolytic treatment should be prescribed; candidates for neurosurgical intervention should be identified. The early course of patients with stroke may be dominated by medical complications and all need close observation and appropriate intervention. This supportive approach is paramount and aimed at preventing secondary brain damage. Physiotherapists and speech therapists play vital roles at this stage. For example, failure to detect risk of aspiration leads to pneumonia, this leads to hypoxia, which causes secondary brain damage, and this equates to a more challenging rehabilitation task. It should be noted that 40% of patients deteriorate after admission to hospital – mostly due to systemic factors. It should also be realized that the care pathway starts at home, the usual place of stroke, and includes all triage up to and including a stroke unit. As early as possible admission into a specialized environment is desirable. Senior medical staff virtually always take lead responsibility for clinical care and commonly lead interdisciplinary teams. In this role they should promote clinical governance and coordinate goal-orientated treatment and discharge planning for individual patients.

## Clinical nurse specialist

The clinical nurse specialist (CNS) is a senior nurse with specific knowledge and experience in the management of patients following stroke. Their primary role is as an educational resource for the team, the patient and their families. This role includes keeping the nursing staff up to date on evidence-based practice in stroke care, leading on development of stroke-related protocols and assisting in health promotion and prevention. On admission, the CNS will meet with the patient and their family and will provide written and/or verbal information on their situation, as appropriate. They act as the patient's advocate throughout their hospital stay and often continue to review the patient following discharge to identify ongoing issues or concerns. Their role after discharge includes providing the patient and carer with information on support groups and making referrals to outside agencies as required.

## Physiotherapy

Physiotherapists may be described as movement specialists, with training in anatomy, kinesiology and biomechanics. During their assessment they observe efficiency, speed, coordination, timing and ease of movement as patients perform functional tasks. Using their knowledge of efficient movement principles they compare patients' movement with perceived normal patterns. This allows the therapist to identify barriers to movement.

Following stroke, a number of impairments may influence the patient's ability to perform functional activities. These include weakness, alterations in tone, sensory loss, reduced balance mechanisms, reduced coordination, fatigue and cardiovascular deconditioning. A painful or subluxed shoulder, altered perception of verticality (pushing) and neglect can also occur. Once identified, these problem areas form the basis of the treatment. Using guided exercises and skilled handling, the physiotherapist aims to allow the patient to repeatedly practise functional tasks, as part of a goal-directed rehabilitation programme. Repeated practice is thought to drive neuroplastic changes (Dobkin, 1998; Turton, 1998; Nundo and Friel, 1999), improve strength and endurance, and aid return to independent living.

Treatment will vary depending on the objective findings (including severity of impairments and level of activity and participation) and on the priorities highlighted by the patient. However, for gains to be made, therapy must be active and context-specific (Dobkin, 1998). Early therapy may focus on practice of bed mobility, regaining sitting balance, facilitating use of the upper limb in functional tasks and standing. Walking is often identified as a main goal and there is evidence that hemiplegic patients can step before regaining standing balance (Kriker et al, 2000), which would support early walking. Recently the use of treadmill training with body weight support has therefore been advocated in retraining gait (Kendrick et al, 2001); however, this has largely been researched in chronic stroke patients. Literature supports the use of the static bike in the more able patient to improve endurance and cardiovascular fitness, but again, this has largely been studied in chronic stroke patients

(Holt et al, 2001). In a subacute and chronic cohort, constraint-induced movement therapy has been advocated to facilitate recovery of activity in the upper limb (Taub et al, 1997; Miltner et al, 1999; Van der Lee et al, 1999). Controversy still surrounds the mechanisms of recovery, i.e. restraint or prolonged periods of practice. This has not been investigated in the acute patient. However, it is suggested that learned non-use occurs early following stroke and that upper limb intervention should commence after seven days (Turton and Pomeroy, 2002). Causes of pushing in stroke remain unclear (Bailey and Leivseth, 2000; Karnath et al, 2000) but have been associated with poorer functional outcomes. There is little written about the treatment of 'pushing' patients, but therapy may focus on reorientating the patient to midline, encouraging them to lie on their non-hemiplegic side while in bed, and reducing over-activity.

During the assessment process, objective measures are taken using measures validated for stroke if possible (RCP, 2000; ACPIN guidelines). Use of objective measures allows identification of changes in the patient's condition to ensure that treatment is targeted effectively.

Following assessment the physiotherapist will liaise with others to recommend appropriate positioning and handling techniques, and methods for assisting the patient to move, transfer and walk if appropriate. These recommendations should be documented as a baseline where all team members can easily refer to them and are updated as the patient progresses.

## Occupational therapy

The role of the occupational therapist (OT) is to assess how the physical, social and psychological effects of stroke impact on the individual's functional ability and their family or significant others. From here the aim is to facilitate the patient's participation in meaningful occupations, this is the core of OT. Trombly (1995) defines occupations as 'the ordinary and meaningful things that people do everyday'.

The process starts with the therapist taking a detailed history of the patient's home situation, physical home environment, social/family networks, work and leisure interests and their roles and responsibilities. The intention of this initial interview is to establish what the patient's lifestyle was before the stroke and enable the therapist to focus on individual priorities. Lifestyle issues are often categorized in three main areas: self-care (e.g. personal washing and dressing, showering/bathing, feeding and using the toilet), productivity (e.g. meal preparation, shopping, maintaining the home environment, working or caring for children/family) and leisure (how the individual enjoys spending free time). If the patient is unable to give this information due to significant language or cognitive deficits, then the information will be gained from other sources, such as family or friends.

Once a premorbid history is established, the OT will assess the patient carrying out a familiar activity or routine, for example, eating a meal or getting dressed. During the observation the OT will assess how motor, sensory, cognitive and perceptual impairments may be impacting on the individual's performance. For example, how left-sided neglect or inattention impacts upon the patient's ability to attend to food on the left side of the plate when eating, or to find the sleeve in their clothing when getting dressed. Both interpersonal and intrapersonal skills will be assessed. Interpersonal skills are those involved in interaction with others, for example, communication skills. Intrapersonal skills are based on individual feelings and attitudes, for example, confidence and adjustment to disability. It is important to identify the strengths and skills during assessment in order to establish the patient's potential to relearn or use techniques and strategies to compensate for their difficulties. For example, does the patient have insight into their problem, which enables them to learn to look to the left side when eating or dressing?

In the acute stage following stroke the OT is most likely to use treatment approaches aimed at restoring function by engaging the patient in meaningful and purposeful occupation, as opposed to purely teaching compensation strategies. Several factors will determine use of approach, such as ability to engage in rehabilitation and previous level of functional independence. OTs use several intervention strategies, including compensations such as adapted methods of doing, adaptive equipment and environmental adaptations (Fisher, 2001). When a compensatory approach is used, the emphasis is on the patient being able to perform the task as independently as possible, within the context of their residual disability.

The OT specific standardized assessments such as the Assessment of Motor and Process Skills (AMPS) and the Canadian Occupational Performance Measure (COPM) (Trombly, 1997) can be used to quantify change in occupational performance and patient satisfaction with performance.

Following the initial interview and baseline functional assessment the OT can then work with the other members of the team to set treatment goals around the patient's identified priorities.

## Speech and language therapy

The speech and language therapist (SLT) is responsible for the assessment and management of speech, language and swallowing difficulties following stroke. The SLT assessment includes a neurological examination of the cranium including evaluation of range, symmetry, strength, speed and coordination of oropharyngeal musculature.

Assessment of dysphagia will, if appropriate, include trialling food and drink of differing consistencies and may also include evaluation of the effectiveness of postural techniques, swallowing manoeuvres or sensory stimulation. Assessment will also take into account the patient's cognitive abilities, insight and ability to comply with advice regarding swallow safety.

The deficits associated with dysarthria and dysphonia include altered respiratory support for phonation, voice quality, oro-motor function, articulation, resonance, rate of speech, prosodic features and speech intelligibility. Difficulties highlighted in assessment will be targeted in SLT sessions via exercises, which aim to improve orofacial symmetry, increase speed and coordination of movement and strengthen orofacial musculature. Techniques used include passive and active oromotor exercises, and breath support and voice exercises. Robertson (2001) showed that a programme of therapy targeted at orofacial muscle movement and articulation proved to be effective in improving speech intelligibility in dysarthric patients who were at least 4 weeks post stroke. In addition, it is important to maintain and facilitate the best use of the patient's retained motor speech skills. This includes practising the use of compensatory strategies to increase intelligibility, for example, slowed rate of speech or increased articulatory effort.

Patients with aphasia may present with difficulties in perception, comprehension and expression of language through both verbal and written modalities. These difficulties can be present at any level, from single words, to sentences, to social conversation and high level reading and writing tasks. Evaluation by the SLT will include formal and informal assessment of specific language impairments and the resulting limitations on functional comprehension and communication.

The literature remains controversial regarding the effectiveness of SLT for patients with aphasia. There are no randomized controlled trials; however, many single case studies and case series have shown therapy to be effective (Whurr et al, 1992; Robey, 1994, 1998; Katz and Wertz, 1997; Greener et al, 1999)

The overall aim of SLT is to enable the patient with aphasia to regain communicative autonomy. The aims of therapy will depend upon the problems identified by assessment. At the level of impairment the aims will be to restore language function by specifically addressing the areas affected and reducing the linguistic deficit. Areas to be targeted may include use of grammar and pragmatics, semantics, reading and auditory comprehension, single word spelling, written grammar or phonological output.

With regard to a patient's limitations of activity and participation, the SLT enables the patient to compensate for their difficulties by providing alternative communication strategies. Use of these strategies should facilitate the effectiveness of retained communication skills. For example, if a patient is unable to communicate their needs verbally but is able to recognize pictures or read single words they may be able to use some form of communication chart. Additional alternative communication methods include use of yes/no systems, self-cueing, gesture or writing. The patient's ability to use strategies will depend on their level of language impairment (particularly comprehension), their motivation, insight, and cognitive, visual and physical abilities. The SLT will also be responsible for educating staff and family in the use of alternative and augmentative communication methods.

Aphasia or dysarthria and the subsequent communication limitations can have a significant effect upon a patient's quality of life and can necessitate psychosocial adjustments for both the patient and their family (Nichols et al, 1996). The SLT will therefore be involved in the facilitation of this adjustment.

## Clinical neuropsychology

Clinical neuropsychology is focused on brain behaviour relationships following brain damage. In the context of stroke, the clinical neuropsychologist is responsible for assessing, monitoring and managing disorders related to cognition, mood and behaviour. A neuropsychology assessment involves measuring cognitive function using a series of tests that are reliable (i.e. they produce the same result over time) and valid (i.e. they measure what they are designed to measure). Following a stroke an individual may present with impairment of one or more cognitive functions. A full neuropsychological assessment would include an investigation of intelligence, memory, language, visual perception, praxis, executive function and speed and attention.

Modern neuropsychology is based on several fundamental assumptions:

1. it is assumed that there is a high degree of functional specialization within the cerebral cortex
2. that complex cognitive skills are made up of several modules
3. brain damage can selectively disrupt some components of the cognitive process (Cipolotti and Warrington, 1995).

One of the key elements of the neuropsychological assessment is to establish whether an individual is functioning at the same level as prior to their stroke or whether this has changed. Thus, an individual's premorbid level of optimal function needs to be estimated first. This may involve an estimate based on their reading performance on a standard test, as reading skill is known to be resistant to most types of brain damage (e.g. National Adult Reading Test, Nelson and Willison, 1991). Alternatively, premorbid level can be estimated on the basis of educational achievement and occupation. Secondly, the neuropsychological assessment provides evidence for an individual's current level of cognitive functioning. Once these two measures have been obtained they can be compared to establish whether there has been any change from the premorbid level estimated, and also the degree of change that has occurred (i.e. the severity of brain damage).

From the neuropsychological assessment a cognitive profile can be constructed in which a comparison across cognitive tasks can be made. This provides a basis for management and allows for monitoring change across time. Common areas of dysfunction following stroke include memory, speed of processing, problem solving, planning and organization, self-monitoring and emotional liability. With regard to planning and monitoring a rehabilitation programme, a neuropsychological assessment can be helpful in providing information to key questions such as whether a patient's treatment goals are realistic and whether they have the capacity to benefit. Further, a cognitive profile that reflects an individual's strengths and weaknesses can be used to provide information to family and carers that may help to explain current problems and prognosis for the future.

## Nutrition and dietetic service

In a stroke unit the dietician provides expert nutrition support and disease-related nutrition education for patients and staff. Within the National Clinical Guidelines for Stroke (Royal College of Physicians, 2002) and the National Service Framework for Older People (Department of Health, 2001), the importance of nutrition and the dietician as an integral part of the stroke team has been clearly recognized. Nutrition intervention at all stages of stroke care can reduce complications, length of stay, morbidity and mortality and improve a patient's quality of life (Finestone et al, 1995).

It is well documented that malnutrition is a common occurrence in hospital patients. Many patients arrive malnourished on admission and their nutritional status declines during the hospital stay (McWhirter and Pennington, 1994). Up to 50% of patients admitted to stroke units are malnourished (Finestone et al, 1995; Molyneaux, 1996). Stroke patients with a poor nutritional status are more likely to have a poor clinical outcome (Finestone et al, 1995). Aside from dysphagia, stroke patients are at risk of malnutrition for a variety of other reasons, for example, lack of consciousness, cognitive problems and lack of appetite. The nutritional management at the early stage post stroke is vital, as the resulting impact of the metabolic response on the body may result in nutritional depletion and hence poor clinical outcome. In an attempt to detect malnutrition and the risks, all patients should be screened within 48 hours of admission and on a regular basis by appropriately trained personnel, using a validated screening method. Screening is important to identify those patients who would benefit from practical interventions at a ward level and to ensure that those patients at high nutritional risk are referred for dietetic intervention.

Maintaining optimal nutrition and hydration requires close collaboration between medical and nursing teams, speech and language therapy and dietetics (Royal College of Physicians, 2002). Dieticians nutritionally assess patients and devise individualized nutritional care plans to promote optimum nutrition. This can be achieved through a variety of methods, for example, food fortification, nutritional supplement products and nasogastric feeding/gastrostomy feeding. As well as regularly monitoring these patients, the dietician is fundamental in designing enteral feeding protocols for nursing staff to follow.

Dieticians can also offer evidence-based secondary prevention dietary advice to patients and their families and/or carers after a stroke and are actively involved in the education of staff in areas such as diabetes and hypercholesterolaemia.

## Interdisciplinary Working

Successful rehabilitation requires effective communication between all members of the interdisciplinary team, including the patient and family/significant others. The Royal College of Physicians (2000) recommends that clinicians should use a common language and framework in order to communicate and agree rehabilitation aims.

The World Health Organization (WHO, 2001) introduced the International Classification of Function (ICF), a detailed classification system that combines medical and social theory to measure health and some health-related components. The ICF supersedes the International Classification of Impairment, Disability and Handicap (ICIDH) developed by the WHO in 1980. In the ICF, health is defined in terms of human functioning rather than disability. Health is measured in terms of two health domains: body functions and structures (impairments) and activities and participation. Impairment refers to signs or symptoms at a body level such as hemiplegia or dysphagia. Activity refers to what was previously described as a disability, an observed function or behaviour. Activity is concerned with the interaction between the individual and the environment and describes what the person can or cannot do; for example, 'able to transfer from bed to wheelchair with minimal assistance from one person'. The participation level of the model was previously referred to as handicap and relates to the social positions or roles that the person has/had. It describes what the patient does within their social context including areas within which they have limitations; for example, 'able to fulfil role of mother/parent with assistance from nanny daily'.

'The ICF provides all those who work in health related spheres with a common language that assists with communication and integrated working' (World Health Organization, 2001). The ICF is also a scientific coding system that can be used as an outcome measure and for research. Having agreed a framework for terminology the team can then use this in written documentation and daily communication throughout the rehabilitation process.

Communication methods may include a daily handover meeting to enable the nursing staff to report changes, that have occurred in the patient's condition overnight. This ensures prompt medical management of any changes and allows the members of the team to prioritize. It is also important to have a weekly multidisciplinary meeting where all members of the team can provide feedback on patients' progress and establish discharge plans and priorities for treatment. Sharing of knowledge by each team member allows for a more holistic understanding of the patient's condition and will facilitate more realistic treatment interventions, taking into account all physical and cognitive deficits. Team members will meet to set goals for the patients. Case conferences or family meetings may be indicated to facilitate effective communication with patients' families regarding progress and discharge planning.

# Interdisciplinary Treatment

Following admission the patient is assessed by all members of the team. The RCP guidelines (1999) recommend that a multidisciplinary assessment using a formal procedure or protocol should be undertaken and documented within 24–48 hours of admission. The results of these assessments are the foundation for goal setting and treatment. For simplicity the rehabilitation process has been split in to two stages: (i) preventing secondary complications and (ii) the rehabilitation process. In practice these are a continuum.

Integrated care pathways (ICP) have been widely researched and their use is supported in many clinical areas. An integrated care pathway may be used to guide the patient's journey through the process of post-stroke rehabilitation. The Royal College of Physicians (2000) recommend using care pathways to organize and deliver care to this patient group. A care pathway is a document that maps what should occur during a specific episode of patient care (Playford et al, 1997). ICPs should be patient-centred and should be developed by all members of the interdisciplinary team involved with patients' care (Coffey et al, 1992; Layton, 1993). They provide a time-related framework for implementation of guidelines based on available evidence regarding the management of all stages of post-stroke care.

## Preventing secondary complications

In the acute stage following stroke, the interdisciplinary team will often be focused on achieving and maintaining medical stability, therefore promoting neural protection and preventing secondary complications. Secondary complications following stroke include chest infections, deep vein thrombosis, pressure area formation, joint stiffness and loss of muscle length. The risk of tissue breakdown is assessed by the nursing staff, and is documented using the waterlow score. If risk is identified a specific pressure relief mattress will be used (Professional Nurse, 1991). The physiotherapist and nursing staff work in close liaison to optimize the patient's positioning in bed and establish an appropriate positioning regime. Little evidence exists as to the optimal positioning after stroke. However, the Royal College of Physicians Guidelines (2000) state that patients should be positioned to minimize the risk of contractures, respiratory complications, shoulder pain and pressure sores. The use of taping, collar and cuffs or slings has been advocated in some instances of shoulder pain or subluxation. However, the literature surrounding their use remains inconclusive (Morley et al, 2002; Turner-Stokes and Jackson, 2002). Best practice is seen as careful handling and positioning.

Another risk to tissue viability is incontinence. Incontinence following stroke is multifactorial, including impairments of memory, communication and mobility. Nursing staff will assess each patient's bladder and bowel function on admission, and will review on a weekly basis. In addition to pressure areas, the potential consequences of incontinence include bladder infections and falls associated with attempting to access the bathroom urgently. Incontinence can have a significant impact on an individual's ability to benefit from rehabilitation and therefore goals to manage incontinence are paramount. Continence charts will be implemented as early as possible, aiming to establish the patient's current patterns. Toileting programmes such as being offered a bottle or being taken to the bathroom 2-hourly will be introduced as necessary. Medications and suppositories may also be used to regularize bowel movements.

Respiratory complications are assessed by the physiotherapist, in conjunction with the nursing and medical teams. Reduced level of alertness, dysphagia, immobility and hemi-respiratory muscle weakness can predispose to chest complications. The physiotherapist may use manual techniques and positioning to aid secretion clearance and prevent atelectasis (Hough, 2001) but sitting the patient out as early as possible should be advocated. Early assessment of swallow function will decrease the risk of chest infection due to aspiration. Dysphagia is common after stroke, occurring in 45–60% of patients (Barer, 1989; Smithard et al, 1996; Daniels et al, 1998). The features indicative of dysphagia and/or aspiration include dysphonia, dysarthria, drooling, abnormal volitional cough, abnormal gag reflex, wet voice post swallow, and coughing or choking on swallowing (Daniels et al, 1998; Warms and Richards, 2000).

The traditionally used assessment of gag reflex has been shown to be unreliable and insensitive as the sole indicator of swallowing function in stroke patients (Bleach, 1993; Davies et al, 1995; Daniels et al, 1998). Therefore patients are initially screened for dysphagia by medical staff or specifically trained nursing staff, using a locally agreed dysphagia screening tool which will include assessment of the indicative features described. Following failure of a screening assessment, patients will be placed 'nil by mouth', prior to further evaluation by a speech and language therapist, as recommended by the Royal College of Physicians Clinical Guidelines for Stroke (1999).

Where indicated the SLT will complete a full evaluation of oromotor and swallow function. Bedside assessment has been shown to have reduced specificity and sensitivity in detecting aspiration (Leder & Espinosa, 2002; Warms & Richards, 2000). Therefore, in cases where further objective measurement is indicated, a videofloroscopic examination (VFS) may be appropriate. VFS is seen as the 'gold standard' in objective dysphagia assessment, as it can detect and reveal the extent and cause of aspiration. In addition, during the VFS, the SLT can evaluate the effectiveness of various techniques in alleviating pharyngeal pooling, penetration or aspiration. VFS has been shown to have improved intra-rater reliability (Scott et al, 1998; McCullough et al, 2001). In the management of dysphagic stroke patients, the aim is to prevent aspiration and to re-establish the safest and most efficient method of swallowing for that individual. The safest option for some patients may be to remain 'nil by mouth' owing to a significant risk of aspiration. Alternatively they may be restricted to modified textures of food and/or fluid to reduce the risk of aspiration. The dietician may advise on additional oral or enteral nutritional supplementation for these patients in order to meet their nutritional requirements.

Specific postures or manoeuvres for swallowing may be introduced, for example, chin tuck, head turn or effortful swallow (Logemann, 1998). Nursing staff will be responsible for ensuring that patients receive the recommended texture of food and drink. They will provide assistance and/or supervision for eating and drinking, ensuring that safe swallowing guidelines are followed. Exercises designed to improve the strength, symmetry and coordination of specific oropharyngeal musculature may also be introduced. These include tongue base strengthening exercises and hyo-laryngeal elevation exercises (Logemann, 1998). Where the patient is unable to maintain adequate oral nutrition, the Royal College of Physicians Guidelines (1999) recommend that a nasogastric (NG) or percutaneous endoscopic gastrostomy (PEG) tube be considered.

If the patient is unable to maintain a seated position independently, the physiotherapist and occupational therapist should assess the patient for a suitable seating system. Assessment for appropriate seating is carried out by observing the patient's postural alignment (Pope, 2002; Turner, 2002). Optimal seating provides enough postural support to maintain alignment of head and trunk and to equalize weight bearing, while challenging the patient to remain upright against gravity thereby encouraging return of activity and postural adjustments. In the early stages a chair with recline or tilt in space facilities may be required if the patient is unable to maintain a seated position against gravity. As the patient improves, their level of support will be reduced. Specialist pressure-relieving cushions are provided to prevent skin breakdown in the immobile patient. Seating tolerance should be increased slowly, depending on the patient's level of alertness and fatigue. The OT, physiotherapist and nursing staff will liaise closely to ensure that a regular programme for sitting out of bed on a daily basis is established.

## Ongoing rehabilitation

For rehabilitation to be effective and relevant to the patient it must be functional and goal orientated, and the patient must have the opportunity for repeated practice. Areas of activity and participation often focused upon in early rehabilitation include the ability to sit, stand, transfer, and walk, to complete personal care activities, meal and drink preparation and to communicate needs. Examples of these areas will be discussed in the case illustration. At later stages in the rehabilitation process more complex and high level activities will be addressed, including return to work and leisure, outdoor mobility, access to public transport and reading and writing.

The priorities for rehabilitation will be set in consultation with the patient, family and members of the interdisciplinary team. Goals will be set on completion of assessments and are used to direct treatment interventions. A goal is a specific measurable statement that reflects the anticipated actions and needs of a person to perform a desired outcome. It refers to the identification of and an agreement of a target which the patient, therapist or team will work towards over a specific period of time (RCP, 2000). Goals are set to measure outcomes of treatment and the patient's performance, to gain a consistent approach to patient care and to improve quality of reha- bilitation through more effective targeting of intervention and monitoring of effects. They also provide a way of planning and doc- umenting progress. Goals must follow a number of requirements. They must be relevant, motivating and express what the patient hopes to accomplish. They should be positively defined and expressed in behavioural terms. They need to be explicit and com- monly understandable (Schut and Stam, 1994). Goals should be written with a positive focus on function and activity rather than impairment and should be written in a way that the patient can understand. For example 'Paul will feed himself independently using a spoon in his right hand' as opposed to 'Paul will have increased range of movement and strength in his right arm'.

It is important to have a system in place for specifying and reg- ularly reviewing the goals for each patient. Action plans relating to a patient's care can also be set before goals related to functional tasks. Establishing the patient's long-term goal enables the team to focus the treatment and discharge plan, and to set short-term goals appropriate to the patient's needs and wishes. Patient-oriented goals can be a challenge in the acute phase when the patient may not be medically well, may not have insight into their condition and func- tional limitations and may not be able to express their needs and wishes effectively. In these cases it may be appropriate to liaise with the patient's family and others. Functional, patient-oriented goals will often cross disciplines and therefore should be set as a team. For example, in aiming to cook a meal the goal will incorporate cognitive, physical and communication skills. The goal may there- fore include elements from all team members as to how a patient will achieve that goal including how much assistance, supervision or prompts will be required. The goals can then be upgraded when achieved by reducing the level of assistance required by the patient or by increasing the complexity of the task. When goals are patient- oriented, focused on function and made explicit to the patient they can be motivating for patient, family and staff. They can also ensure that care and rehabilitation are coordinated so that all members of the team, including the patient and their family, are working towards an agreed outcome.

Early discharge planning provides the team with a focus for their treatment plans and goals. Discussions regarding appropriate discharge destination should therefore commence as soon as all members of the team have completed their assessments in conjunction with the patient and their significant others. The choice of discharge destination will be dependent on severity of stroke, physical and cognitive status, ability to participate in rehabilitation, potential for change and exercise tolerance. Prompt referral to appropriate agencies including social services and community rehabilitation teams will facilitate a timely and seamless discharge for the patient.

## Case illustration

The following case study is an illustration of interdisciplinary working in practice.

### Medical history

Ms A was admitted to hospital via the Accident and Emergency Department following sudden onset of right-sided weakness and difficulty speaking. Clinical examination suggested an extensive left MCA syndrome, confirmed on neuroimaging. Underlying risk factors included hypertension, non-insulin-dependent diabetes mellitus (NIDDM) and smoking.

### Social situation

Ms A is a previously independent lady who is married with two teenage children and works full time in a supermarket. In her leisure time she enjoys spending time with her family. She also likes reading crime novels, doing crosswords, baking and sewing.

*contd . . .*

## Impairments on admission

- Severe right-sided weakness
- Reduced balance mechanisms
- Sensory loss and altered perception of midline orientation
- Severe expressive and receptive dysphasia
- Oropharyngeal dysphagia
- Bladder and bowel dysfunction
- Reduced insight to difficulties
- Reduced reasoning and problem solving
- Impaired short-term memory

## Activity and participation on admission

- Dependent on maximal assistance for bed mobility
- Dependent on use of a hoist and the assistance of two people to transfer from bed to chair
- Dependent on maximal aid of one person to sit
- Dependent on a NG tube for nutrition and hydration
- Dependent on a catheter for bladder management
- Dependent for all personal care
- Unable to communicate basic needs
- Cognitive difficulties impacting upon functional tasks
- Unable to work, pursue leisure activities or perform role as a mother

## Intervention and rehabilitation

Following assessment, areas for priority of intervention were identified. In the initial stages Ms A was unable to identify her priorities due to communication and cognitive impairments. She had limited functional activity and was dependent for all care. Intervention was therefore targeted at prevention of secondary complications including respiratory complications, shoulder pain and chest infections. She was placed nil by mouth because of the risk of aspiration and received regular physiotherapy treatment for her chest status. Her seating needs were assessed to allow early sitting out to aid chest care. Positioning regimes whilst in bed were documented. Ms A's

*contd . . .*

family were informed of her progress and were consulted with regard to treatment planning. The allocated keyworker acted as the advocate for Ms A and her family.

The following limitations of activity and participation were addressed during the rehabilitation stage.

• Dependent on maximal assistance for bed mobility

Early therapy sessions included practice of bed mobility, such as rolling and getting from lying to sitting. Repeated practice of the task occurred initially with the aid of the therapist or nurses with the level of support being reduced as Ms A improved. This helped in the recruitment and strengthening of trunk muscles. Before practice of these tasks began, the physiotherapist addressed muscle imbalance, muscle shortening and realignment of joints to enable the optimal recruitment of muscles.

• Dependent on maximal aid of two people to sit

Initially Ms A required the maximum aid of two people to sit on the side of the bed. Daily sitting practice encouraged recruitment of trunk activity. As sitting balance improved support was reduced. Reaching for objects or engaging Ms A in functional tasks (e.g. washing face) was used to recruit more trunk activity.

• Dependent on use of a hoist and the assistance of two people to transfer from bed to chair

Ms A was initially stood with the assistance of four people from a high plinth. Standing up against gravity hopes to encourage the recruitment of extensor activity throughout the body. While in standing position Ms A was encouraged to practise functional tasks to encourage the stimulation of postural adjustments. As activity was regained the number

*contd . . .*

of people required to stand Ms A reduced. Standing was progressed to stepping with the support of three. This was progressed to walking short distances with physical assistance from the therapists.

• Dependent on a NG tube for nutrition and hydration

Bedside assessment and subsequent videofluoroscopic examination of swallowing revealed moderate oropharyngeal dysphagia. Soft diet and moderately thickened fluids were introduced with specific instructions to carry out chin tuck for drinking. Nursing staff were informed of the safe swallowing guidelines and Ms A's family were educated regarding these techniques. Oro-motor exercises were carried out regularly by staff and family to increase range and strength of movement of tongue, tongue base and lip seal.

• Dependent on a catheter for bladder management

Ms A was commenced on a regular toileting regime. She was initially offered the bedpan in bed every 2 hours. As she progressed she was able to indicate her need for the toilet using a picture communication chart. As mobility improved she began to use a commode, transferring with assistance.

• Dependent for all personal care

Practice of personal care began in supported sitting, as it was too demanding for Ms A to concentrate on washing and maintaining her posture. She was inattentive to her right and required verbal and physical cues to attend to her right side. Initially her right upper limb was placed supported on a table in front to encourage her to attend to it. As movement returned she was encouraged to incorporate it into tasks with assistance from the therapists. As mobility improved Ms A was progressed to performing some aspects of her personal care in supported standing.

*contd . . .*

• Unable to communicate basic needs

In order to enable Ms A to regain some degree of communicative autonomy alternative communication methods were trialled. Through repetition in a variety of functional situations, including personal care and toileting, she developed the ability to communicate her basic daily needs via a picture communication chart. Use of more advanced alternative communication was limited by Ms A's visual perceptual difficulties and reduced attention, concentration and memory.

• Cognitive difficulties impacting upon functional tasks

Due to reduced ability to plan and organize self-care tasks, Ms A required full set up of items before initiating the activity. As she made progress, set up was reduced and prompting was used to encourage Ms A to plan and organize her personal care. In addition, reduced concentration and attention necessitated short treatment periods with reduced distractions within the environment. Lack of insight to difficulties and reduced problem solving had some impact upon Ms A's ability to use strategies to compensate for her physical impairments. Awareness was increased through concrete feedback on performance within functional activities. Problem solving was assisted by breaking all activities down into small manageable steps. The task difficulty was slowly increased to allow more complex problems to be attempted as she improved.

• Unable to work, pursue leisure activities or perform role as a mother

During the acute stage of rehabilitation it was not appropriate to address these issues. Therefore continued rehabilitation was recommended due to Ms A's potential for further progress. She was referred to a local inpatient rehabilitation unit where she received 4 months of intensive rehabilitation. The areas would be addressed in further rehabilitation.

*contd . . .*

## Activities and participation on discharge

- Dependent on moderate assistance of one person for bed mobility
- Transferring through stand with moderate aid of two people
- Able to walk short distances with the maximum aid of three
- Able to sit unsupported on bedside with supervision
- Eating a soft diet and drinking thin fluids with chin tuck and supervision
- Continent of bladder and bowels
- Able to wash top half in sitting with aid of one person to incorporate right upper limb
- Communicating basic needs verbally with occasional use of pictures and/or gestures
- Able to use basic strategies to aid problem solving and attention
- Able to sustain attention for 30-minute sessions without prompting

## Summary

Unfortunately, a recipe for acute multidisciplinary care following stroke cannot be given, as each patient presents with a different range of impairments and different levels of activity and participation. In addition, patients will all identify individual priorities for intervention according to their own needs, backgrounds, experience and culture. However, as this chapter has aimed to outline, there are key themes within our assessment and treatment of this client group. Firstly, successful rehabilitation relies on effective teamworking, which is based on a shared language and shared understanding of the needs of the patients. Communication is central to such a coordinated approach. Professional roles may overlap with blurring of traditional boundaries. This facilitates a holistic and consistent approach to patient care and avoids unnecessary duplication within assessment and documentation. Secondly, by setting functional goals with patients and their families, an appropriate, patient-led plan of care and rehabilitation will be instigated. Goals that are identified by the patient as relevant and motivating will facilitate their participation in the rehabilitation process. In addition, successful multidisciplinary rehabilitation requires an environment where 24-hour management of patients provides opportunities for patients to have repeated practice of functional rehabilitation activities relevant to the goals identified. This provides the most appropriate environment to facilitate recovery.

# References

Bailey MJ, Leivseth L (2000) The pusher syndrome in elderly stroke patients. *British Journal of Therapy and Rehabilitation* **7**: 11–16.

Barer DH (1989) The natural history and functional consequences of dysphagia after hemispheric stroke. *Journal of Neurology, Neurosurgery and Psychiatry* **52**: 236–41.

Bleach NR (1993) The gag reflex: a retrospective analysis of 120 patients assessed by videofluoroscopy. *Clinical Otolaryngology* **18**: 303–7.

Cipolotti L, Warrington EK (1995) Neuropsychological assessment. *Journal of Neurology, Neurosurgery and Psychiatry* **58**: 654–5.

Coffey RJ, Richards JS, Renert CS, Leroy SS, Schoville RR, Baldwin PJ (1992) An introduction to critical care pathways. *Quality Management Healthcare* **1**: 45–5.

Daniels SK, Brailey K, Priestly DH, Herrington LR, Weisberg LA, Foundas AL (1998) Aspiration in patients with acute stroke. *Archives of Physical and Medical Rehabilitation* **79**: 14–19.

Davies AE, Kidd D, Stone SP, MacMahon J (1995) Pharyngeal sensation and gag reflex in healthy subjects. *Lancet* **345**: 487–8.

Department of Health (2001) *National Service Framework for Older People.* Department of Health, London.

Dobkin BH (1998) Activity dependent learning contributes to motor recovery. *Annals of Neurology* **44**: 158–60.

Fisher A (2001) *Assessment of Motor and Process Skills*, 3rd edn. Three Star Press, USA.

Finestone HM, Greene-Finestone LS, Wilson ES, Teasell RW (1995) Malnutrition in stroke patients on the rehabilitation service and at follow up. *Archives of Physical Medicine and Rehabilitation* **77**: 340–5.

Freeman M, Proctor-Childs T (1998) Vision of Team Working: The Realities of an Interdisciplinary Approach. *British Journal of Therapy and Rehabilitation* **5**: 616.

Greener J, Enderby P, Whurr R (1999) Speech and language therapy for aphasia following stroke (Cochrane Review). In: *The Cochrane Library*, Issue 4. Update Software, Oxford.

Holt R, Kendrick C, McGlashan K, Kirker S, Jenner J (2001) Static bicycle training for functional mobility in chronic stroke. *Physiotherapy* **87**: 257–60.

Hough A (2001) *Physiotherapy in Respiratory Care: An Evidenced-based Approach to Respiratory and Cardiac Management.* Chapman and Hall, Cheltenham.

Johnson J (1995) Achieving effective rehabilitation outcomes: does the nurse have a role? *British Journal of Therapy and Rehabilitation* **2**: 113–18.

Karnath HO, Ferber S, Dichgans J (2000) The origin of contraversive pushing. *Neurology* **55**: 1298–304.

Katz RC, Wertz RT (1997) The efficacy of computer-provided reading treatment for chronic aphasic adults. *Journal of Speech, Language & Hearing Research* **40**: 493–507.

Kendrick C, Holt R, McGlashan K, Jenner RJ, Kirker S (2001) Exercising on a treadmill to improve functional mobility in chronic stroke patients. *Physiotherapy* **87**: 261–5.

Kirker SGB, Simpson DS, Jenner JR, Wing AM (2000) Stepping before standing: hip muscle function in stepping and standing balance after stroke. *Journal of Neurology, Neurosurgery and Psychiatry* **68**: 458–64.

Layton A (1993) Planning individual care with protocols. *Nursing Standard* **8**: 32–4.

Leder SB, Espinosa JF (2002) Aspiration risk after stroke: comparison of clinical examination and fibreoptic endoscopic examination of swallowing. *Dysphagia* **17**: 214–18.

Logemann JA (1998) *Evaluation and Treatment of Swallowing Disorders*, 2nd edn. Pro-Ed, Texas.

McCullough GH, Wertz RT, Rosenbek JC, Mills RH, Webb WG, Ross KB (2001) Inter- and intra-judge reliability for videofluoroscopic swallowing evaluation measures. *Dysphagia* **16**: 110–18.

McWhirter VP, Pennington CR (1994) Incidence and recognition of malnutrition in hospitals. *British Medical Journal* **308**: 945–8.

Miltner WH, Bauder H, Sommer M, Dettmers C, Taub E (1999) Effects of constraint-induced movement therapy on patients with chronic motor deficits after stroke: a replication. *Stroke* **30**: 586–92.

Molyneaux H (1996) Malnutrition following brain injury. *European Journal of Neurology* **3**: 45.

Morley A, Clarke A, English S, Helliwell S (2002) Management of the subluxed low tone shoulder. *Physiotherapy* **88**: 208–15.

Nelson HE, Willison J (1991) *The National Adult Reading Test*, 2nd edn. NFER-Nelson, Windsor, UK.

Nichols F, Varchevker A, Pring T (1996) Working with people with aphasia and their families: an exploration of the use of family therapy techniques. *Aphasiology* **10**: 767–81.

Nundo RJ, Friel KM (1999) Critical plasticity after stroke: implications for rehabilitation. *Revue Neurologique* **155**: 713–17.

Playford ED, Rossiter D, Werrin DJ, Thompson AJ (1997) Integrated care pathways: evaluating inpatient rehabilitation in stroke. *British Journal of Therapy and Rehabilitation* **14**: 97–102.

Pope P (2002). Posture management and special seating. In: Edwards S, ed. *Neurological Physiotherapy; a problem solving approach*, 2nd edn. Churchill Livingstone, Edinburgh: 189–217.

Robertson S (2001) The efficacy of oro-facial and articulation exercises in dysarthria following stroke. *International Journal of Language and Communication Disorders* **36**: 292–7.

Robey R (1994) The efficacy of treatment for aphasic persons: a meta-analysis. *Brain & Language* **47**: 582–608.

Robey R (1998) A meta-anaysis of clinical outcomes in the treatment of aphasia. *Journal of Speech Hearing Research* **41**: 172–87.

Roper N, Logan W, Tierney A (1980) *The Elements of Nursing*. Churchill Livingstone, Edinburgh.

Royal College of Physicians (1999, 2000, 2002) *National Clinical Guidelines for Stroke* (www.rcplondon.ac.uk).

Schut HA, Stam HJ (1994) Goals in rehabilitation teamwork. *Disability and Rehabilitation* **16**: 223–6.

Scott A, Perry A, Bench J (1998) A study of interrater reliability when using videofluoroscopy as an assessment of swallowing. *Dysphagia* **13**: 223–7.

Smithard DG, O'Neill PA, Parks C, Morris J (1996) Complications and outcome after acute stroke. Does dysphagia matter? *Stroke* **27**: 1200–4.

Stroke Unit Trialists Collaboration (1997) How do stroke units improve patient outcomes? A collaborative systematic review of the randomized trials. *Stroke* **28**: 2139–44.

Stroke Unit Trialists' Collaboration (2000) Organised inpatient (stroke unit) care for stroke. *Cochrane Database Systematic Review* (2): CD000197.

Taub E, Wolf SL (1997) Constraint induced movement techniques to facilitate upper extremity use in stroke patients. *Topics in Stroke Rehabilitation* **3**: 38–61.

Trombly CA (1995) Occupation, purposefulness and meaningfulness as therapeutic mechanisms. *American Journal of Occupational Therapy* **49**: 960–72.

Trombly CA (1997) *Occupational Therapy for Physical Dysfunction*, 4th edn, 45–8. Williams and Wilkins, Baltimore.

Turner C (2002) Posture and seating for wheelchair users; an introduction. *British Journal of Therapy and Rehabilitation* **8**: 24 –8.

Turner-Stokes L, Jackson D (2002) Shoulder pain after stroke: a review of the evidence base to inform the development of an integrated care pathway. *Clinical Rehabilitation* **16**: 276–98.

Turton A (1998) Mechanisms for recovery of hand and arm function after stroke: a review of evidence from studies using non-invasive investigative techniques. *British Journal of Occupational Therapy* **61**: 359–64.

Turton A, Pomeroy V (2002) When should upper limb function be trained after stroke? Evidence for and against early intervention. *Neuro-Rehabilitation* **17**: 215–24.

Van der Lee JH, Wagenaar RC, Lankhorst GJ, Vogelaar PT, Deville WL, Bouter LM (1999) Forced use of the upper extremity in upper extremity chronic stroke patients. *Stroke* **30**: 2369–80.

Warms T, Richards J (2000) Wet voice as a predictor of penetration or aspiration in oropharyngeal dysphagia. *Dysphagia* **15**: 84–8.

Waterlow J (1991) A Policy that Protects, the Waterlow Pressure Sore Prevention/Treatment Policy. *Professional Nurse* **6**: 258–64.

Whurr R, Lorch MP, Nye C (1992) A meta-analysis of studies carried out between 1946 and 1988 concerned with the efficacy of speech and language therapy treatment for aphasic patients. *European Journal of Disorders of Communication* **27**: 1–18.

World Health Organization (2001) *International Classification of Functioning Disability and Health (ICF)*. WHO, Geneva.

# 3

# The Impact of the Disease: A Medical View

*Richard Greenwood*

## Introduction

Stroke, or vascular brain injury, is a major cause of death, disablement and loss of quality of life. It is the commonest life-threatening neurological condition and single cause of severe disablement in people living at home (Harris, 1971; Martin et al, 1988; Wolfe, 2000), comprising 20–30% of people with chronic conditions, who alone account for 80% of health-care costs (Hoffmann et al, 1996). Some 70–75% of strokes are ischaemic in origin, 10–15% are the results of primary intracerebral haemorrhage, about 5% are due to subarachnoid haemorrhage and the rest are undefined. Large artery disease and cardiac embolism account for 20% and 25% of ischaemic strokes respectively, and lacunar strokes for 25% (Petty et al, 1999).

Stroke has significant impact on families, carers, and health and social service professionals and resources managing acute and long-term needs. It accounts for 5% of acute medical admissions. In England and Wales each year about 110,000 people have their first stroke and 30,000 have further strokes, so that at any one time there are 25–35 patients with stroke as their primary diagnosis in an average general hospital (Pearson et al, 1994; Rudd et al, 1999; Department of Health, 2001). The cost and impact of stroke are likely to rise as the population ages and its cost-effective management is of general importance.

## Mortality, Incidence and Prevalence

Most epidemiological studies have been done in white populations in industrialized countries, where stroke accounts for about 10% of all deaths (about 60,000 per annum in England and Wales) and follows myocardial infarction and cancer as the third most common cause of death. Nearly 90% of victims are over 65 years of age. Mortality from stroke has been decreasing over the last 50 years, though probably less so recently (Feigin et al, 2003), for reasons that are unclear. The 1-month overall case-fatality rate is 20–25% after first stroke, 10–15% after cerebral infarction and 40–50% after primary intracerebral or subarachnoid haemorrhage (Bamford et al, 1990a; Stewart et al, 1999). Most deaths in the first 7 days after stroke are caused by neurological complications, most between 7 and 30 days are the result of the complications of immobility, whilst cardiovascular disease is the commonest cause of death subsequently (Bamford et al, 1990b; Dennis et al, 1993). The overall 5-year survival rate is 40–60% (Dennis et al, 1993; Lindmark and Hamrin, 1995; Wilkinson et al, 1997).

Stroke incidence is now not clearly decreasing, probably due to ageing of the population, and is about 2 per 1000 or about 500 cases per year per 250,000 population. In South London in 1995 and 1996, the incidence for first ever stroke (representing about 75% of all acute strokes) was found to be 1.3 per 1000 population, 1.1 per 1000 white people and 2.6 per 1000 black people, the latter comparable to the highest rates worldwide (Stewart et al, 1999). About 75% of patients are over 65 years, 10% under 55, and each year in England and Wales stroke occurs in about 10,000 people under 55 and 1000 people under 30. About 30% of patients recover but about 50% require some assistance.

Prevalence of stroke survivors in populations surveyed over 20 years ago in Australia, Finland and Copenhagen (Christie, 1981; Sorensen et al, 1982; Aho et al, 1986) has been estimated at 5–8 per 1000 population or 50–70 per 1000 population over the age of 65, and is similar in studies since 1990 (Feigin et al, 2003). Residual disability is seen in 50–75% of cases (Bonita et al, 1997; O'Mahony et al, 1999). About 75–80% of cases regain at least indoor walking, 55% can live independently, 40–50% are unable to walk outdoors, 70% have at least some difficulties walking and do not regain normal age-related walking speed, 35% are significantly disabled, and 10–15% require daily help with personal care, but 40–50% return to work or use public transport independently.

Recent longitudinal studies have found that at 6–12 months post stroke, 25–30% of survivors have difficulty with bathing or using stairs, 30–40% are depressed (10–15% severely so), 50% need help with either housework, meal preparation or shopping, and a similar number lack a meaningful social, recreational or occupational activity during the day (Thorngren et al, 1990; Kauhanen et al, 1999; Mayo et al, 2002). Clearly, these problems may be ameliorated by support in the community, and increased community reintegration correlates with better quality of life at 6 months (Mayo et al, 2002). This support needs to be available rather than highly skilled, but there is evidence to suggest that its sole provision by a spouse risks a low quality of life in the patient at 1 year (Kauhanen et al, 2000). Between 3 and 12 months and 5 years post stroke, motor performance and functional independence deteriorate in up to 40% of survivors, largely due to ageing and co-morbidity rather than recurrent stroke (Viitanen et al, 1988; Lindmark and Hamrin, 1995; Wilkinson et al, 1997). To what extent this deterioration can be prevented has not been determined, although day hospital care has been shown to prevent deterioration in activities of daily living in the frail elderly (Forster et al, 2000).

## Outcomes After Stroke

It is important that these consequences of stroke are mapped on to a more general classification of the consequences of disease. An initial classification of the observable consequences of a 'health condition' was provided by the World Health Organization (WHO) International Classification of Impairments, Disabilities, and Handicaps (ICIDH) in 1980. The ICIDH assumed dysfunction and classified abnormality, or behaviour in ill health, and thus automatically disenfranchized people with disablement (Oliver, 1990). This is corrected in the new WHO International Classification of Functioning, Disability and Health (2001), which classifies behaviours in health which may be altered by ill health. *Disabilities* become *Activities* which may be 'limited' whilst *Handicap* becomes *Participation* which may be 'restricted'. *Activities* classify function at the level of the person alone, *Participation* classifies the extent of a person's involvement and engagement in life's situations and social roles. The *Impairment* dimension continues to classify loss or abnormality of body structures and physiological or psychological functions and *Contextual factors* are added as a fourth dimension.

These may be either *Personal*, for example, age, gender, personality and premorbid characteristics that may play a role in the experience of disablement, or *Environmental* – comprising aspects of the physical and social world extrinsic to the individual. These factors are determinants of *Participation* but also may modify *Activities* or *Impairments* and are themselves potentially mutable and targets for intervention.

The disablement phenomena of the WHO classifications do not include measures recording aspects of an individual's judgement of their life experience. As Fuhrer (1994) has emphasized, if the goal of rehabilitation is to 'make life worth living' then measures of life quality and subjective well-being and its component concepts, and the way in which they relate to *Impairments*, *Activities* and *Participation* need considerable investigation. This will make it possible to justify interventions, particularly late post stroke, which generate less obviously useful changes than cost or care containment. Reliable measurement of these separate dimensions is important because change as a result of treatment is most likely to be detected by measurement of the dimension in which the treatment is delivered, and because changes in one dimension may not necessarily be reflected linearly by changes in another. For example, after head injury subjective quality of life correlates inversely with severity of injury (Brown and Vandergoot, 1998), whilst after spinal injury a measure of life satisfaction correlates with measures of *Participation* but not the extent of paralysis (*Impairment)* or dependence in activities of daily living (*Activities*) (Fuhrer et al, 1992).

In summary therefore, the impact (Figure 3.1) for an individual of a disease or illness such as stroke involves observable functional abilities that comprise health status on the one hand, the individual's view of their well-being or life quality on the other, and the personal and environmental contexts in which the disease occurs (Figure 3.1A). The extent of impact changes with time and interventions (Figure 3.1B). The interaction of these multidimensional constructs is usually complex and non-linear (Wade, 1996), so that to obtain an adequate representation of the effects of the disease, and thus the usefulness and timeliness (Whyte, 1994) of an intervention, measurement of outcome in several dimensions is necessary. A former emphasis on measures of physical self-care, omitting those relating to well-being, satisfaction, quality of life and return to work or leisure activities (Seale and Davies, 1987), is being replaced by an understanding that quality of life after stroke is severely affected both physically and emotionally, often reflecting the degree to which victims lack rehabilitative and social support (Kauhanen et al, 2000; O'Connell et al, 2001; Mayo et al, 2002).

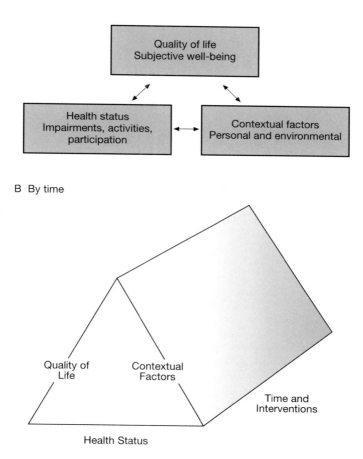

**Figure 3.1** Comprehensive assessment of the consequences and outcome of a health condition or disease at any single instant (A) and longitudinally (B).

# Evolution of Impact

Recovery of impairments and functional independence is most rapid in the first days and few weeks post stroke, when resolution of penumbral ischaemia, oedema and mass effects, and diaschisis are likely to play important roles in clinical improvement (Furlan et al, 1996; Seitz et al, 1999). Later neurological improvements are associated with ipsi- and contra-lesional reorganization of use-dependent neuronal networks (described in Chapter 1), and functional independence is further increased by learning adaptive techniques and modification of environmental contextual factors. These changes may not continue to occur in the absence of community or outpatient rehabilitation, when deterioration may occur and was seen for example in the 'no treatment group' in the Northwick Park outpatient study (Smith et al, 1981).

Apart from adverse personal and environmental contextual factors, mortality, neurological recovery, dependency and resource use are particularly predicted by the severity of the initial neurological insult. Signs reflecting brainstem dysfunction, by direct involvement or mass effect, including decreased conscious level, a conjugate gaze palsy, severe bilateral weakness, and an abnormal pattern of respiration are associated with a high early mortality (Tijssen et al, 1991; Henon et al, 1995). In the Oxford Community Stroke Project, after total anterior circulation infarction (TACI), mortality and independence at 1 year were 60% and 40% respectively, compared with 10–15% and 60–70% respectively, after partial anterior circulation infarction (PACI) and lacuna infarction (LACI) (Bamford et al, 1990a, 1991). Smith and Baer (1999) have shown that of TACI survivors, 77% achieved independent sitting balance over a median time of 11 days, 50% standing balance (median time 44 days), 36% achieved 10 supervised steps (median time 88 days), and 30% a supervised 10-metre walk (median time 113 days). After PACIs and LACIs the majority of patients achieved all these goals within 3 weeks; length of stay was five to six times longer after a TACI. Predictors of better outcome after a TACI, apart from age, social back-up and low body temperature, remain uncertain (Jorgensen et al, 1999).

Other clinical features may be used to assist in the prediction of impact. Urinary incontinence, present as a result of stroke in 40% of patients at 7–10 days and 10% at 2 years, is associated with adverse long-term outcomes (Patel et al, 2001). The absence of hand grip at 14 days predicts a non-functional arm at 3 months (Heller et al, 1987); severe dysphasia on admission predicts severe dysphasia at 6 months in 40% of survivors (Pedersen et al, 1995); and persisting visual neglect at 6 months is predicted by severe visual neglect and the presence of anosognosia at 2–3 days post stroke (Stone et al, 1992). The additional use of modern imaging techniques (e.g. Shelton and Reding, 2001; Baird et al, 2001) or motor-evoked potentials (e.g. Pennisi et al, 1999), particularly very early post stroke when clinical predictors are less reliable may provide additional information, although their usefulness will be limited by availability. Data of this sort help expectation to match experience and guide clinical practice and discussion about goal setting, transfer to further rehabilitation and discharge planning; they should be used to predict expected floors and ceilings of attainment rather than exact longer-term targets.

In parallel and over 1–2 years or longer, a grieving process occurs in the patient and allows adaptation to loss of premorbid competencies; it may require facilitation to enable reasonable quality and satisfaction with life. Failure to support patients adapting to role loss and change is likely to increase depression which, with cognitive problems, contributes to a reduction in leisure and social activities to a degree far greater than predicted by levels of physical function (Pound et al, 1998; Clark and Smith, 1999; Burton, 2000; O'Connell et al, 2001).

At the same time, adjustments are necessary among family members (Holbrook, 1982) if they are to interact effectively with the patient despite the physical, cognitive, emotional and behavioural consequences of stroke, all recognized potential sources of major burden in the spouse and other informal carers (Anderson et al, 1995; Scholte op Reimer et al, 1998; Han and Haley, 1999; Low et al, 1999; Smout et al, 2001). Informal carers should be recognized as an important resource: they enable patients to remain in the community (Hancock and Jarvis, 1994), their support is likely to facilitate patient outcomes (Anderson et al, 1995), and levels of depression in the patient are greater in those who feel poorly supported (Morris et al, 1991).

These adaptive changes, both in patient and carer, are potential targets for interventions but are seldom seen to be so. Controlled studies that show, for example, an increase in activity and participation in the patient may have difficulty showing life quality or adaptive changes (Logan et al, 1997). Formal support for carers is

difficult to obtain but there is evidence to suggest that carer adjustment is increased by education and counselling (Evans et al, 1988)
or by training in social problem-solving skills (Grant et al, 2002),
clinical interventions not generally utilized in the trials of family
support that have failed to show functional or psychological benefit
(Christie and Weigall, 1984; Friedland and McColl, 1992; Forster
and Young, 1996; Dennis et al, 1997; Lincoln et al, 2003). Focused
prescription of clinical intervention for carers might be assisted by
reliable prediction of carers at risk of later strain (Blake et al, 2003).

## Resource Implications

Acutely after stroke, assessment of disordered systemic and neurological physiological homeostasis, with a view to its maintenance,
is a priority, in parallel with investigations, particularly imaging, to
establish the nature of the pathological insult. Levels of blood pressure, temperature, oxygen saturation, hydration and glycaemia need
to be rapidly established with a view to manipulation as required.
This must be followed by a more detailed assessment of the patient's
neurological and cognitive status, their mood, behaviour, and extent
of immobility, continence, and pain and discomfort. These multidisciplinary assessments of impairment underpin the formulation of
an integrated care plan and individualized goals, and also, with premorbid personal and contextual factors in mind, enable a long-term
functional prognosis and, in discussion with the patient and family
as possible/appropriate, the start of realistic discharge plans and
arrangements for ongoing collaborative and goal-orientated support
and rehabilitation in the community.

This type of organized care requires a defined geographical area
in the hospital and a coordinated interdisciplinary team to reduce
mortality and dependence at 1 year (Stroke Unit Trialists
Collaboration, 1997, 2000). However, organizational change, at
least in the UK, is difficult and the most recent National Sentinel
Stroke Audit for England and Wales from the Royal College of
Physicians (RCP) in London for 2001–2 found that only 36% of
admitted patients spent any time, and only 27% the majority of their
time, on a stroke unit, whilst 55% of cases spent the majority of their
stay on a general ward (Table 3.1). Thus in the UK many patients are
still not subject to timely assessment and treatment of their major
functional deficits, even as inpatients. In addition, European studies
indicate that outcome is poorer in the UK (Wolfe et al, 1999, 2001).

**Table 3.1.** Examples of compliance with process standards in the RCP National Sentinel Stroke Audit 2001/2

| Standard | *Compliance with standard* |
|---|---|
| Screening for swallowing disorders (not gag reflex) has been specifically recorded in the first 24 hours | 64% |
| The patient has been assessed by a physiotherapist within 72 hours of admission (or of stroke if the stroke occurred in hospital) | 59% |
| There is evidence that the patient's mood has been assessed | 52% |
| There is a plan to promote urinary continence | 63% |
| Individualized goals include reference to areas of higher level functioning (e.g. leisure pursuits, driving, returning to work) by the time of discharge | 24% |
| The carer's needs for support were assessed separately | 41% |
| A home visit was performed | 73% |
| The patient has received rehabilitation since discharge if required | 65% |
| There is evidence of a review at approximately 6 months (4–8 months) following discharge from inpatient therapy of mood, psychological needs and social reintegration (e.g. work, leisure, social support) | 51% |

There is also a considerable shortfall in assessment, let alone treatment, of their psychosocial needs, even at follow-up, and only 26% of stroke units had sessional allocation for a clinical psychologist.

This makes dismal reading and must contribute to longer-term functional deficit and a reduction in life quality in stroke survivors in the community. Thus a Norwegian study (Indredavik et al, 1997) has shown functional benefit even 5 years after acute and rehabilitation stroke unit treatment compared with treatment on a general ward, 35% versus 18% ($p = 0.006$) of patients respectively still being at home. The implication of the Stroke Unit Trialists Collaboration data, reiterated by the Department of Health's *National Service Framework (NSF) for Older People* (2001), is that organized care, and thus compliance with the simple standards of the RCP Sentinel Audit, can be achieved by reallocation of resources and improved governance, at no overall additional cost to health and social care, especially if combined with early supported discharge (Anderson et al, 2000; Early Supported Discharge Trialists,

2000). That the low compliance with standards of adequate care results at least partly from difficulties in organizational change, is illustrated by the high compliance in the RCP Audit with actions which take one person 2 minutes to undertake, for example the prescription of antithrombotic (91%) or lipid-lowering (79%) agents at discharge. Successful modification of organizational behaviour is likely to increase the provision of organized care and significantly reduce the impact of stroke in the UK.

# References

Aho K, Reunanen A, Aromaa A, Knekt P, Maatela J (1986) Prevalence of stroke in Finland. *Stroke* **17**: 681–6.

Anderson C, Mhurcha CN, Rubenach S, Clark M, Spencer C, Whinsor A (2000) Home or hospital for stroke rehabilitation? Results of a randomised controlled trial. I: Health outcomes at 6 months. *Stroke* **31**: 1024–31.

Anderson GS, Linto J, Steward-Wynne EG (1995) A population-based assessment of the impact and burden of care giving for long term stroke survivors. *Stroke* **26**: 843–9.

Baird AE, Dambrosia J, Janket S-J et al (2001) A three-item scale for the early prediction of stroke recovery. *Lancet* **357**: 2095–9.

Bamford J, Sandercock P, Dennis M, Burn J, Warlow C (1990a) A prospective study of acute cerebrovascular disease in the community: the Oxfordshire Community Stroke Project – 1981–86. 2. Incidence, case fatality rates and overall outcome at one year of cerebral infarctions, primary intracerebral and subarachnoid haemorrhage. *Journal of Neurology Neurosurgery and Psychiatry* **53**: 16–22.

Bamford J, Dennis M, Sandercock P, Burn J, Warlow C (1990b) The frequency, causes and timing of death within 30 days of first stroke: the Oxfordshire Community Stroke Project. *Journal of Neurology Neurosurgery and Pychiatry* **53**: 824–9.

Bamford J, Sandercock P, Dennis M, Burn J, Warlow C (1991) Classification and natural history of clinically identifiable subtypes of cerebral infarction. *Lancet* **337**: 1521–6.

Blake H, Lincoln NB, Clarke DD (2003) Caregiver strain in spouses of stroke patients. *Clinical Rehabilitation* **17**: 312–17.

Bonita R, Solomon N, Broad JB (1997) Prevalence of stroke and stroke-related disability. *Stroke* **29**: 866–7.

Brown M, Vandergoot D (1998) Quality of life for individuals with traumatic brain injury: comparison with others living in the community. *Journal of Head Trauma Rehabilitation* **13**: 1–23.

Burton CR (2000) Living with stroke: a phenomenological study. *Journal of Advanced Nursing* **32**: 301–9.

Christie D (1981) Prevalence of stroke and its sequelae. *Medical Journal of Australia* **2**: 182–4.

Christie D, Weigall D (1984) Social work effectiveness in two-year stroke survivors: a randomised controlled trial. *Community Health Studies* **8**: 26–32.

Clark M, Smith D (1999) Psychological correlates of outcome following rehabilitation from stroke. *Clinical Rehabilitation* **13**: 129–40.

Dennis MS, Burn JPS, Sandercock AG, Bamford JM, Wade DT, Warlow CP (1993). Long term survival after first ever stroke; the Oxfordshire Community Stroke Project. *Stroke* **24**: 796–800.

Dennis M, O'Rourke S, Slattery J, Staniforth T, Warlow C (1997) Evaluation of a stroke family careworker: results of a randomised controlled trial. *British Medical Journal* **314**: 1071–6.

Department of Health (2001) *National Service Framework for Older People.* DoH, London. (http://www.doh.gov.uk/nsf/olderpeople.htm).

Early Supported Discharge Trialists (2000) Services for reducing duration of hospital care for acute stroke patients. In: *The Cochrane Library.* Update Software, Oxford.

Evans RL, Matlock A-L, Bishop DS, Stranahan S, Pederson C (1988) Family intervention after stroke: does counselling or education help? *Stroke* **19**: 1243–9.

Feigin VL, Lawes CMM, Bennett DA, Anderson CS (2003) Stroke epidemiology: a review of population-based studies of incidence, prevalence, and case-fatality in the late 20th Century. *Lancet Neurology* **2**: 43–53.

Forster A, Young J (1996) Specialist nurse support for patients with stroke in the community: a randomised controlled trial. *British Medical Journal* **312**: 1642–6.

Forster A, Young J, Langhorne P for the Day Hospital Group (2000) Medical day hospital care for the elderly versus alternative forms of care. In: *The Cochrane Library.* Update Software, Oxford.

Friedland JF, McColl M (1992) Social support intervention after stroke: results of a randomised trial. *Archives of Physical Medicine and Rehabilitation* **73**: 573–81.

Fuhrer MJ (1994) Subjective well-being: implications for medical rehabilitation outcomes and models of disablement. *American Journal of Physical Medicine and Rehabilitation* **73**: 358–64.

Fuhrer MJ, Rintala DH, Hart KA, Clearman R, Young ME (1992) Relationship of life satisfaction to impairment, disability, and handicap among persons with spinal cord injury living in the community. *Archives of Physical Medicine and Rehabilitation* **73**: 552–7.

Furlan M, Marchal G, Viader F, Derlon J-M, Baron J-C (1996) Spontaneous neurological recovery after stroke and the fate of the ischaemic penumbra. *Annals of Neurology* **40**: 216–26.

Grant JS, Elliott TR, Weaver M, Bartolucci AA, Giger JN (2002) Telephone intervention with family caregivers of stroke survivors after rehabilitation. *Stroke* **33**: 2000–65.

Han B, Haley WE (1999) Family care giving for patients with stroke. Review and analysis. *Stroke* **30**: 1478–85.

Hancock R, Jarvis C (1994) *The Long Term Effects of Being a Carer*. HMSO, London.

Harris AI (1971) *Handicapped and Impaired in Great Britain. Part 1*. Office of Population Censuses and Surveys. HMSO, London.

Heller A, Wade D, Wood VA, Sunderland V, Hewer RL, Ward E (1987) Arm function after stroke: measurement and recovery over the first three months. *Journal of Neurology Neurosurgery and Psychiatry* **50**: 714–19.

Henon H, Godefroy O, Leys D et al (1995) Early prediction of death and disability after acute cerebral ischaemic events. *Stroke* **26**: 392–8.

Hoffman C, Rise D, Sung H-Y (1996) Persons with chronic conditions. Their problems and costs. *JAMA* **276**: 1473–9.

Holbrook M (1982) Stroke: social and emotional outcome. *Journal of the Royal College of Physicians London* **116**: 100–4.

Indredavik B, Slørdahl SA, Bakke F, Rokseth R, Håheim LL (1997) Stroke unit treatment. Long-term effects. *Stroke* **28**: 1861–6.

Jorgensen HS, Reith J, Nakayama H, Kammersgaard LP, Raaschou HO, Olsen TS (1999) What determines good recovery in patients with the most severe strokes? The Copenhagen stroke study. *Stroke* **30**: 2008–12.

Kauhanen M-L, Korpelainen JT, Hiltunen P et al (1999) Post stroke depression correlates with cognitive impairment and neurological deficits. *Stroke* **30**: 1875–80.

Kauhanen M-L, Korpelainen JT, Hiltunen P, Nieminen P, Sotaniemi KA, Myllylä VV (2000) Domains and determinants of quality of life caused by brain infarction. *Archives of Physical Medicine and Rehabilitation* **81**: 1541–6.

Lincoln NB, Francis VM, Lilley SA, Sharma JC, Summerfield M (2003) Evaluation of a stroke family support organiser. A randomised controlled trial. *Stroke* **34**: 116–21.

Lindmark B, Hamrin E (1995) A five-year follow-up of stroke survivors: motor function and activities of daily living. *Clinical Rehabilitation* **9**: 1–9.

Logan PA, Ahern J, Gladman JRF, Lincoln NB (1997) A randomised controlled trial of enhanced social services occupational therapy for stroke patients. *Clinical Rehabilitation* **11**: 107–13.

Low J, Payne S, Roderick P (1999) The impact of stroke on informal carers: a literature review. *Social Science and Medicine* **49**: 711–25.

Martin J, Meltzer H, Elliot D (1988) OPCS Surveys of disability in Great Britain Report 1. In: *The Prevalence of Disability Among Adults*. Office of Population Censuses and Surveys, HMSO, London.

Mayo NE, Wood-Dauphinee S, Côté R, Durcan L, Carlton J (2002) Activity, participation, and quality of life 6 months post stroke. *Archives of Physical Medicine and Rehabilitation* **83**: 1035–42.

Morris PL, Robinson RG, Raphael B, Bishop D (1991) The relationship between the perception of social support in post-stroke depression in hospitalised patients. *Psychiatry* **54**: 306–16

National Sentinel Stroke Audit 2001/02. Royal College of Physicians, London (http://www.rcplondon.ac.uk/college/ceeu/strokeconciseauditreport.pdf).

O'Connell B, Hanna B, Penney W, Pearce J, Owen M, Warelow P (2001) Recovery after stroke: a qualitative perspective. *Journal of Quality Clinical Practice* **21**: 120–5.

Oliver M (1990) *The Politics of Disablement.* MacMillan, London.

O'Mahony PG, Thomson RG, Dobson R et al (1999) The prevalence of stroke and associated disability. *Journal of Public Health Medicine* **21**: 166–71.

Patel M, Coshall C, Rudd AG, Wolfe CDA (2001) National history and effects on 2-year outcome of urinary incontinence after stroke. *Stroke* **32**: 122–7.

Pearson MG, Littler J, Davies PD (1994) An analysis of medical workload – evidence of patient to specialist mismatch. *Journal of the Royal College of Physicians London* **28**: 230–4.

Pedersen PM, Jorgensen HS, Nakayama H, Raaschou HO, Olsen TS (1995) Aphasia in acute stroke: incidence, determinants, and recovery. *Annals of Neurology* **38**: 659–66.

Pennisi G, Rapisarda G, Bella R, Calabreze V, Noordhourt AM de, Delwaide PJ (1999) Absence of response to early transcranial magnetic stimulation in ischaemic stroke patients. Prognostic value for hand motor recovery. *Stroke* **30**: 2666–70.

Petty GW, Brown RD, Whisnant JP, Sicks JD, O'Fallon WN, Wiebers DO (1999) Ischaemic stroke subtypes. A population-based study of incidence and risk factors. *Stroke* **30**: 2513–16.

Pound P, Gompertz P, Ebrahim S (1998) A patient-centred study of the consequences of stroke. *Clinical Rehabilitation* **12**: 338–47.

Rudd AG, Irwin P, Lowe D, Wade D, Morris R, Pearson MG (1999) The national sentinel audit for stroke: a tool for raising standards of care. *Journal of the Royal College of Physicians London* **33**: 460–4.

Scholte op Reimer WJM, de Hann RJ, Pijnenborg JMA, Limburg M, van den Bos GAM (1998) Assessment of burden in partners of stroke patients with the sense of competence questionnaire. *Stroke* **29**: 373–9.

Seale C, Davies P (1987) Outcome measurement in stroke rehabilitation research. *International Disability Studies* **9**: 155–60.

Seitz RJ, Agari NP, Knorr U, Binkofski F, Herzog H, Freund H-J (1999) The role of a diaschisis in stroke recovery. *Stroke* **30**: 1844–50.

Shelton F de NAP, Reding MJ (2001) Effect of lesion location on upper limb motor recovery after stroke. *Stroke* **32**: 107–12.

Smith D, Goldenberg E, Ashburn A et al (1981) Remedial therapy after stroke: a randomised controlled trial. *British Medical Journal* **282**: 517–20.

Smith MT, Baer GD (1999) Achievement of simple mobility milestones after stroke. *Arch Phys Med Rehabil* **80**: 442–7.

Smout S, Koudstaal P, Ribbers G, Janssen W, Passchier J (2001) Struck by stroke: a pilot study exploring quality of life and coping patterns in younger patients and spouses. *International Journal of Rehabilitation Research* **24**: 261–8.

Sorensen PS, Boysen G, Jensen G, Schnohr P (1982) Prevalence of stroke in a district of Copenhagen. The Copenhagen City Heart Study. *Acta Neurologica Scandanavica* **66**: 68–81.

Stewart JA, Dundas R, Howard RS, Rudd AG, Wolfe CDA (1999) Ethnic differences in incidence of stroke: prospective study with stroke register. *British Medical Journal* **318**: 967–71.

Stone SP, Patel P, Greenwood RJ, Halligan PW (1992) Measuring visual neglect in acute stroke and predicting its recovery: the visual neglect recovery index. *Journal of Neurology, Neurosurgery and Psychiatry* **55**: 431–6.

Stroke Unit Trialists Collaboration (1997) How do stroke units improve patient outcomes? A collaborative systematic review of the randomized trials. *Stroke* **28**: 2139–44.

Stroke Unit Trialists' Collaboration (2000) Organised inpatient (stroke unit) care for stroke. *Cochrane Database Systematic Review* (2): CD000197.

Thorngren M, Westling B, Norrving B (1990) Outcome after stroke in patients discharged to independent living. *Stroke* **21**: 236–40.

Tijssen CC, Bento PN, Schulte MD, Anton CM, Leyten MD (1991) Prognostic significance of conjugate eye deviation in stroke patients. *Stroke* **22**: 200–2.

Viitanen M, Fugl-Meyer KS, Bernspång B, Fugl-Meyer AR (1988) Life satisfaction in long-term survivors after stroke. *Scandanavian Journal of Rehabilitation Medicine* **20**: 17–24.

Wade DT (1996) Epidemiology of disabling neurological diseases: how and why does disability occur? *Journal of Neurology Neurosurgery and Psychiatry* **61**: 242–4.

Wade DT, Langton Hewer R (1987) Functional abilities after stroke: measurement, natural history and prognosis. *Journal of Neurology Neurosurgery and Psychiatry* **50**: 177–82.

Whyte J (1994) Toward a methodology for rehabilitation research. *American Journal of Physical Medicine and Rehabilitation* **73**: 428–35.

Wilkinson PR, Wolfe CDA, Warburton FG et al (1997) A long-term follow-up of stroke patients. *Stroke* **28**: 507–12.

Wolfe CDA (2000) The impact of stroke. *British Medical Bulletin* **56**: 275–86.

Wolfe CDA, Tilling K, Beech R, Rudd AG; for the European BioMED study of stroke care group (1999) Variations in death and disability from stroke in western and central Europe. *Stroke* **30**: 350–6.

Wolfe CDA, Rudd AG, Dennis M, Warlow C, Langharne P (2001) Taking acute stroke care seriously. *British Medical Journal* **323**: 5–6.

World Health Organization (1980) *ICIDH: International Classification of Impairment, Disabilities, and Handicaps. A Manual of Classification Relating to the Consequences of Disease*. WHO, Geneva.

World Health Organization (2001) *The International Classification of Functioning, Disability and Health – ICF*. WHO, Geneva.

# 4

# The Impact of the Disease: A Personal View

*Robert McCrum*

I was 42 years old when I suffered my stroke, a 'right-side haemor-rhagic infarct'. Paralysed on my left side and unable to walk, I was confined to hospital for 3 months, then spent about a year recovering, slowly getting myself back into the world. At the time it happened I had virtually no knowledge of the affliction that is 'the commonest life-threatening neurological condition and single cause of severe disablement in people living at home', but overnight I became an instant expert, and so did my wife and immediate family circle. This is something, I think, that doctors are inclined to overlook – the effect of the patient's stroke on his or her immediate community. As for myself, once I was out of danger, it became part of my long recovery to find out all I could about my condition. In that respect I was fortunate to find myself being treated at the National Hospital in Queen Square, one of the world's great centres for neurological illness, and to have as my consultants Richard Greenwood and Andrew Lees, who are both outstanding in their respective fields.

No one can argue with Dr Greenwood's impressive list of stroke statistics. It makes chilling reading, and it brings back to me yet again the awesome finality of stroke as a killer and a disabler. But what I want to focus on in this chapter is what I see as the missing dimension to the medical profession's account of stroke, i.e. the patient's feelings. As I've said on countless occasions, stroke is an earthquake at the centre of who we are, and it is our emotions – assuming we survive – upon discovering that our body is no longer responsive to routine everyday instructions that I believe to be as worthy of consideration as the medical condition.

These are the many unmentionables of stroke: the rage and the depression, the crying and the fear of the night; the sense of shame and indignity that afflicts the stroke sufferer, young or old. When I was in Queen Square, I found myself wanting to tell health-care workers what it felt like to feel suddenly on the scrap heap of life, but because my speech was slurred and my mind confused, I felt unable to articulate such thoughts. I certainly wanted stroke doctors to know that the medical profession's honourable refusal to commit itself to an interpretative prognosis with very many stroke patients can be a source of immense anger and frustration. Also, more positively, I wanted to record my opinion that, if my example was to be trusted, the brain seems to be an astonishingly resilient organ, and one capable, in certain circumstances, of remarkable and surprising regeneration. Even today, I still find new pathways opening up between my brain and previously paralysed parts of my left side.

Leaving aside the physical specifics to which stroke doctors rightly direct their professional attention, the human cost of stroke is profound but because this can really only be appreciated by those who have experienced an 'insult to the brain', it remains beyond the reach of most doctors' understanding. Take, for instance, the simple matter of the fatigue that follows a stroke. The word itself fails to do justice to the enfeebling power of post-stroke fatigue. In my case – which I'm sure is typical – the smallest exertion left me wanting to lie down and go to sleep. The muscles on my left side were so weak that to sit in a chair – which I wasn't able to do, even with nurses to help me, for some days – was exhausting.

With fatigue came depression. As Richard Greenwood correctly identified to me at this time, this would be at its worst at the point at which I was just beginning to make progress (the movement of a finger; a waggling toe; a slight but miraculous wrist movement). It was partly to fight depression, and to give myself something positive to think about that I began to make notes for the book that became *My Year Off: Rediscovering Life After a Stroke*. At times, my year off was one of all pervading slowness, of weeks lived one day, even one hour, at a time, and of life circumscribed by quite exasperating new restrictions and limitations. It doesn't matter whether you are young or old (and 20% of all strokes will occur under 40): the experience is the same. The only thing that differs is long-term scale. *My Year Off* became the record of a journey into my personal interior, not I hope a sentimental or self-pitying account, but a work of reportage by a writer who earns his living as a journalist.

Looking back, I think I was fortunate. I was relatively young and fit and though, at first, my recovery seemed incredibly slow, once I began to get movement back in my left leg and left arm, I continued to make small, incremental improvements long after I had been told my condition would cease to get better. Nonetheless, and although I adopted a positive attitude towards my fate fairly early on in my convalescence, I can say with hindsight that the 'grieving process' for my old life lasted, slowly lessening in intensity, for at least 5 years. Indeed, not until my second daughter, Isobel, was born, nearly 5 years after the stroke, did I begin to feel at peace with my place in the world, and reconciled to my fate.

My post-stroke world is not ideal. But I'm grateful to be alive, and recognize that even if I was fully fit I would still be dissatisfied. There are things I would like to be able to do, but can't. I'm still vulnerable to irrational bursts of frustrated anger, which is upsetting to those, like my wife, who have to live with them. But, partly through the writing of my book, and the voluntary stroke rehabilitation work to which this has led, I have become able to lead a normal and fulfilling life. I know I have been fortunate: there are thousands of stroke sufferers all over Britain for whom stroke has been followed by the three Ds: Disability, Divorce, Despair, often linked to redundancy in all senses. As I wrote at the onset: this is an affliction that has an emotional cost. To tackle it requires emotional willpower. In *My Year Off,* the account of my experience, I listed some Do's and Don'ts for the convalescent stroke-sufferer. Under Do's, I listed the following:

1. Try alternative therapies, like acupuncture
2. Find out as much as you can about your illness
3. Take the initiative
4. Accept help from friends and relatives
5. Trust your body
6. Give yourself Time
7. Meet and talk with other stroke-sufferers (Different Strokes).

My personal Don'ts are simpler and more fundamental:

1. Don't despair
2. Don't imagine you are forgotten
3. Don't surrender.

Now, nearly 8 years later, that sunny July morning of 1995 seems like a strange dream. Sometimes I wake at first light. And I wonder: Did it really happen? But of course it did. All I want to say now is that a stroke is half medical and physical, and half psychological and emotional. It is a frustrating condition to the medical profession, because the usual doctor–patient contract – Diagnosis, Treatment, Cure – doesn't really work with stroke. But just because you cannot see and treat the wound, does not mean that doctors should overlook the pain of it.

## Bibliography

McCrum R (1998) *My Year Off: Rediscovering Life after a Stroke.* Picador, London.

# 5

# Evaluating the Outcome of Rehabilitation Interventions

*Mehool Patel and Anthony Rudd*

## Stroke Outcome

### What is stroke outcome?

The term 'outcome' initially referred to the technical result of a diagnostic procedure or treatment episode. However, this clinical approach was found to be inappropriate for many health service activities, especially for those involving chronic diseases such as stroke. Donabedian therefore suggested the concept of evaluating quality of health care in terms of three separate aspects: the *structure* of the service, the *process* of care and the *outcome* of care. Donabedian's formal definition of outcome was a change in a patient's current and future health status that can be attributed to antecedant health care (Donabedian, 1980). Outcome could be alternatively defined as the overall long-term impact of health interventions both on the population as a whole and on individuals in particular (Stojcevic et al, 1996).

### For whom is stroke outcome being assessed?

An important aspect of research into outcomes of chronic diseases such as stroke is establishing for whom is the outcome being measured and for what purpose (Stojcevic et al, 1996). Is the outcome in question going to be of relevance to the patients, their formal/informal carers, the clinicians, service providers, politicians, or society more broadly? The answer to this question will be vital in establishing the appropriate outcome for any studies or audit of clinical practice. An approach looking at the possible process/outcome measures that could be used by various groups involved with stroke services was suggested by Long in 1995 (Table 5.1). This grid approach does tease out the issues, but one could argue that a multidisciplinary team should work together with common objectives and tools to measure these objectives.

## Tools for assessment of stroke outcomes

Apart from being the third most common cause of death (Murray and Lopez, 1997; Office of National Statistics, 1997), stroke is also the most common cause of adult disability in the Western world (Martin et al, 1989; Mayo et al, 1999). This is because the sequelae of stroke can impact on virtually all human functions: gross and fine motor ability, ambulation, capacity to carry out basic and instrumental activities of daily living, mood, speech, perception and cognition. Moreover, it is different from many other disabling conditions in that the onset is sudden, leaving the individual and the family ill prepared to deal with its sequelae. Hence, due to the chronic and heterogeneous nature of stroke, it is necessary for studies in stroke outcomes to:

(i) Embrace a wider perspective than survival, impairment, recurrence or physical recovery and include broader measures of stroke outcomes, and include disability, handicap and health-related quality of life measures to provide a more holistic measure of stroke outcome.

(ii) Look beyond the short-term outcome and investigate the long-term consequences in population-based studies in order to provide useful baseline information for planners of rehabilitation services and longer-term care, and also for future intervention trials aiming to improve these outcomes. Such long-term studies would help health-care professionals involved in stroke care to balance the potential risks and benefits of treatment options and make rationing decisions if resources are limited (Hankey et al, 2000).

**Table 5.1** For whom is the outcome being measured (Long, 1995)

| Defining group | User/carer | Primary care team | Hospital team | Commissioner |
|---|---|---|---|---|
| Reasons for interest | • At risk of stroke<br>• Has had stroke<br>• Recovery from stroke<br>• Long-term disability | • Responsible for prevention<br>• Diagnosis and referral in acute stage<br>• Long-term care<br>• Pastoral care<br>• Purchasing | • Acute care of patient<br>• Assessment, planning, treatment and evaluation<br>• Rehabilitation<br>• Coordinates care | • Health of population<br>• Allocation of resources<br>• Purchasing<br>• Monitoring<br>• Evaluation |
| Desired outcomes | • Reduced risk of stroke<br>• Early diagnosis and treatment<br>• No complications<br>• Minimal disability and handicap<br>• Good quality of life<br>• Support at all stages | • Low incidence of stroke<br>• Accurate diagnosis and quick transfer to appropriate unit<br>• Good communication, coordination of care<br>• Effective rehabilitation<br>• Patient returns home<br>• Minimal disability<br>• Minimal anxiety and stress | • Effective assessment procedures acceptable to all professionals<br>• No complications<br>• Minimal disability<br>• Good communications with primary care team<br>• Patient and carer satisfied and understand illness<br>• Patient returns home | • Effective health promotion/prevention<br>• Low incidence and prevalence of stroke<br>• Effective treatment<br>• Appropriate length of hospital stay<br>• Appropriate discharge destination<br>• Care coordinated<br>• Cost-effective care package |

contd . . .

**Table 5.1** contd

| Defining group | User/carer | Primary care team | Hospital team | Commissioner |
|---|---|---|---|---|
| Possible outcome measures | • Disability and handicap<br>• Quality of life<br>• Patient satisfaction | • Stroke incidence<br>• Mortality<br>• Time to transfer to hospital<br>• Disability and handicap<br>• Patient satisfaction<br>• Coordinated care | • Mortality<br>• Complication rates<br>• % assessed at 1 week<br>• Incontinence at 1 week<br>• Discharge destination<br>• Disability and handicap<br>• Patient satisfaction | • % hypertensives treated<br>• Incidence, mortality<br>• Length of stay<br>• Disability and handicap<br>• % discharged home<br>• % patients on aspirin<br>• % with key worker<br>• % attending day centre<br>• Stroke register in use |

The concept of broader measures of disease outcomes was globally recognized in 1980 with the development of the *International Classification of Impairments, Disabilities, and Handicaps (ICIDH)* under the auspices of World Health Organization (Wood, 1980). There are various definitions given for these domains of outcome, as described in Table 5.2. This model of illness has recently been revised so that in the new version the emphasis on the personal, social, and physical context has been expanded (WHO, 1999). In the new model, disability is referred to as 'activity' and handicap has become 'participation'. These changes have been made to reflect the need for more neutral, less medically biased terminology. These broader domains of outcomes are essential for the complete assessment of rehabilitation of patients with stroke. It is important to expand the understanding of the effects of stroke on the social roles of these patients in order to gain a greater knowledge of those factors that are instrumental in restricting or enhancing the life activities of stroke survivors (Clarke et al, 1999).

Another distinct but overlapping paradigm that is also relevant for describing the impact of stroke on the individual is health-related quality of life (HRQOL) (Patrick and Deyo, 1989; Bowling, 1995). Increasing a patient's quality of life should be an important target of rehabilitation. It has also been suggested that this may be equated to reducing handicap and that assessments of quality of life and handicap may be more relevant than changes in impairments or disabilities (Ebrahim, 1990). A review of outcome measures in stroke rehabilitation research in 1987 criticized the lack of use of broader measures and suggested that quality of life should be included in future studies (Seale and Davies, 1987). Another review on stroke outcome measures in 174 acute stroke trials, performed between 1955 and 1995, showed that death was recorded in 76%, impairment in 76%, disability in 42% and handicap or HRQOL in only 2% (Roberts and Counsell, 1998). The review also reported that the period of follow-up was often too short to assess the full impact of treatment on the final status of the patient.

## Disability after stroke

Disability is a good indicator of functional outcome and there are several validated tools that can assess disability after stroke (Table 5.2). Most measures of disability take into account essential activities for independent daily living such as walking and eating.

**Table 5.2** Definitions and scales of different domains used in stroke outcomes*

| Outcome | Definitions | Examples of measures available |
|---------|-------------|-------------------------------|
| Impairment | WHO (1999): loss or abnormality of anatomical, physiological or psychological structure or function | Glasgow Coma Scale (consciousness) |
| | | MRC grades of power (motor weakness) |
| | | Motricity Index (motor weakness) |
| | Wade (1992): the immediate consequence of pathology as perceived by the individual; impairment affects actions which in themselves have no meaning | Ashworth Scale (spasticity) |
| | | Behavioural Inattention Test (neglect) |
| | | Frenchay Aphasia Screening Test (aphasia) |
| | | Mini-mental State Examination (cognition) |
| | Duckworth (1992): bits that won't work | Hospital Anxiety and Depression (depression) |
| | | Scandinavian Stroke Scale (severity) |
| | | National Institute of Health Stroke Scale (severity) |
| | | Orgogozo Stroke Scale (severity) |
| Disability or activity | WHO (1999): restriction or lack of ability to carry out activities in an appropriate or normal manner | Barthel Index (BI) |
| | | Katz ADL |
| | | Functional Ambulation Category (FAC) |
| | Wade (1992): the effect pathology or impairment has upon actions which have some meaning to the person | Rivermead activities of daily living (RADL)[†] |
| | | Extended activities of daily living (EADL)[†] |
| | | Instrumental activities of daily living (IADL) |
| | Duckworth (1983): activities that cannot be carried out | Nottingham extended activities of daily living (NEADL)[†] |

*contd . . .*

* Advantages and disadvantages of these scales are well described by Wade (1992) and Bowling (1995).
[†] These scales have been used for both disability and handicap in various studies.

**Table 5.2** contd.

| Outcome | Definitions | Examples of measures available |
|---|---|---|
| Handicap or participation | WHO (1999): disadvantage to given individual, resulting from an impairment or disability that limits or prevents the fulfilment of a role that is normal for that individual<br><br>Wade (1992): the freedom the person has lost due to the pathology; it is judged with reference to the cultural, social, economic and physical environment of the individual<br><br>Duckworth (1992): roles that cannot be performed | Rankin scale (RS)[†]<br>Modified Rankin Scale (MRS)[†]<br>Oxford Handicap Scale (OHS)<br>Mobility Handicap (MH)<br>Glasgow Outcome Scale (GOS)<br>London Handicap Scale (LHS)<br>Frenchay Activities Index (FAI)[†]<br>Reintegration to normal living index (RNLI)<br>Adelaide Activities Profile (AAP)[†] |
| Health-related quality of life (HRQOL) | Kaplan (1995): impact of disease and treatment on disability and daily function<br><br>Greer (1984): physical, emotional and social well-being after diagnosis and treatment | Short-Form 36 (SF-36) and Short-Form 12 (SF-12)<br>Physical health summary score of SF-36 (PHSS)<br>Mental health summary score of SF-36 (MHSS)<br>EuroQol<br>Nottingham Health Profile (NHP)<br>Sickness Impact Profile (SIP)<br>Stroke Specific SIP (SS-SIP)<br>Life satisfaction index (LSI)<br>Visual Analogue Scale (VAS)<br>Social Behaviour Assessment Schedule (SBAS)<br>Ferrans & Powers QOL index (QLI)<br>General Health Questionnaire (GHQ)<br>2-simple questions |

[†] These scales have been used for both disability and handicap in various studies.

Disability remains significantly prevalent for several years following a stroke, with previous studies reporting 8–66% of their sample having some disability (Patel et al, 2001). This variation is due to differences in the design and sample of the studies (Patel et al, 2001). These include variations in time since stroke at which assessments were made, the cross-sectional nature of several studies with patients being observed at different times after stroke, and the numerous outcome measures being used.

Determinants of disability following stroke include (Task Force on Stroke, 1990): demographic factors such as age, impairments (e.g. extent of paralysis, visual or cognitive impairment, urinary incontinence, depression, spasticity and central pain), complications such as pressure sores or urinary tract infections; and co-morbidity such as pre-existing heart or lung disease.

The importance of research into disability after a stroke is highlighted by the recommendation from government institutions such as the UK Department of Health that purchasers of health-care services should identify and monitor indicators of stroke outcome, such as a reduction in disability (Department of Health, 1993). One way may be to enhance community services and include the provision of day hospitals, intermittent respite care and social support centres to minimize handicap and improve HRQOL. The need for improved standards of long-term stroke care, including better community services (intermediate care), have received national recognition by the government of England in its recently published document entitled *National Service Framework for Older People* (Department of Health, 2001).

## Handicap after stroke

Stroke studies have estimated the prevalence of handicap to be between 12–64% (Patel et al, 2001). The reasons for this variation are similar to those mentioned earlier for disability as well as due to the diversity in social structures in different research settings (Patel et al, 2001). Different handicap scales may also explain some of these differences. For example, handicap 1 year after stroke was 12% using the Oxford Handicap Scale in one study (Samuelsson et al, 1996), whereas it was 37% in another using the Frenchay Activities Index (Dijkerman et al, 1996). It is vital to recognize that unlike impairment and disability, handicap is not disease-specific and reflects social, cultural, economic and environmental consequences for the individual that stem from the presence of impairment or disability. It is a good marker for the integration between the effects of disease, medical and rehabilitative therapy, environmental adaptations, formal and informal help, and psychological state. Moreover unlike disability, measurement of handicap is difficult and, as outlined by Wade (1992), there are three major problems in its assessment:

(i) It has to be assessed with reference to specific culturally based expectations of the individual patient, so there is no absolute standard for judging handicap.

(ii) As handicap arises from the interaction between disability and environment, it is also necessary to assess the environment (for example, public attitudes and economic aspects).

(iii) In contrast to disability, which refers to skills and behaviours, handicap cannot be observed directly, and this poses a problem within a 'scientific paradigm'.

Despite these difficulties in assessing handicap, it has important theoretical advantages as an outcome measure (Harwood et al, 1994). By concentrating on the habitual abilities and limitations on someone's life, given their own personal circumstances (for example, their physical environment, wealth, relationships, and availability of aids and equipment), handicap gives a relevant description of the needs for and effectiveness of health and other services (Harwood et al, 1994).

Assessment of handicap becomes particularly relevant in long-term stroke outcomes, especially beyond 1 year after stroke. This is because after 1 year, by which time impairments and disabilities would have stabilized (Wade and Hewer, 1987), improvement in health status might be brought about by various processes of adaptation (Harwood et al, 1997). These include the learning of new skills (as opposed to the recovery of old skills which were lost), psychological adjustment to disability resulting in changes in expectations, alterations in the environment, and the acquisition of aids and appliances. All these processes or changes can be captured well by assessing handicap.

## Health-related quality of life (HRQOL) after stroke

Although widely used in clinical and research settings to assess stroke outcome from a broader perspective, disability and handicap are nevertheless objective tools of stroke outcome. As stated earlier, another domain that is gaining popularity in addressing the impact of stroke subjectively, from a patient's perspective, is health-related quality of life (HRQOL) (Patrick and Deyo, 1989; Bowling, 1995). By examining the relationship between HRQOL with disability and handicap, one can establish whether these objective tools of assessment of stroke outcome are also relevant to patients themselves.

Despite the growing research into HRQOL and its measurement, it is still very rarely measured in routine clinical practice. Barriers to using HRQOL in clinical practice include concerns about cost, feasibility and clinical relevance (Deyo and Carter, 1992). For HRQOL measures to be suitable for clinical use they must be simple, quick to complete, easy to score, able to provide useful clinical data, reliable, valid, appropriate, responsive to change, and able to be interpreted clinically (Higginson and Carr, 2001). HRQOL is difficult to measure because perception of quality of life varies between individuals, and also varies within individuals over time (Lindley et al, 1994).

There have been studies looking at simple questions to assess disability and HRQOL after stroke and thereby provide a minimalist measurement tool to assess outcome in large trials and epidemiological studies after stroke (Lindley et al, 1994; Dorman et al, 2000). These questions assessed dependency and recovery and helped to classify patients into three main categories: dependent, independent but not recovered, and independent and fully recovered. That concept is heavily biased towards physical functional abilities and has several disadvantages (Dorman et al, 2000) including inability to provide a broad and global picture of HRQOL; inability to capture information on outcome in specific domains such as psychological functioning, household maintenance and communication problems; and inability to assess how a treatment improves overall HRQOL. Moreover, a recent study showed that there were significant variations in the sensitivity and specificity of these questions across various European centres (McKevitt et al, 2001). These differences raise questions about how patients interpreted and answered these questions.

## Multidimensional stroke outcomes

Investigating the relationships between disability, handicap and HRQOL is desirable in order to evaluate the perspectives of each of these stroke outcomes with one another as well as to allow us to focus on specific outcome measures (e.g. the Barthel Index) rather than the numerous measures currently used in the vain hope of capturing stroke outcomes. Previous studies (Duncan et al, 1997) indicate that standardized assessment of individuals with stroke must evaluate across the entire continuum of health-related functions, and recommend that measures such as the SF-36 be used in addition to the Barthel Index, which has a ceiling effect and captures only physical functions.

The data and safety monitoring committee for the National Institute of Neurological Disorders and Stroke (NINDS) – Recombinant Tissue Plasminogen Activator – Stroke Trial recommend that a positive result for a single outcome would not provide sufficient evidence of efficacy, but instead suggest measuring four outcomes – Barthel Index, Modified Rankin Scale, Glasgow Outcome Scale, and the National Institute of Health Stroke Scale – and then using a single global statistical test to compare these outcomes simultaneously (Tilley et al, 1996). This is because for many interventions, no single measure of disability can describe all the dimensions of recovery that may be affected by the intervention. Moreover, as there is to date no effective treatment available for stroke which would effectively eliminate the associated handicap and poor HRQOL, it is in fact necessary to assess disability, handicap and HRQOL as primary outcome measures in all stroke studies.

Future studies on stroke outcomes should include long-term follow-up at several time points to determine changes in associations between performance-based measures and HRQOL over time, and larger studies to confirm or refute the associations reported to date. Mortality rates should also be considered in conjunction with the prevalence rates of these domains in order to address the potential confounding situation, whereby a new intervention or process of care for stroke patients may enhance survival but consequently yield more disabled and/or handicapped patients.

## Cost-effectiveness of stroke care

Apart from clinical outcomes, cost-effectiveness of specific interventions is also of paramount importance in stroke. This is best evaluated by a cost-utility analysis which uses a uniform measure in health improvement called quality-adjusted life-year (QALY) (Gold et al, 1996). A QALY is the number of life-years saved adjusted for the quality of these saved life-years with the use of utilities (1 corresponds to optimal health and 0 to death). Hence, it captures both HRQOL and length of life in the same measure. A systematic review of economic evaluation in stroke research reported that: (i) the majority of the studies measured the costs and consequences of interventions only during the hospital stay and there were no studies that had looked at costs beyond a year after stroke; (ii) only one study used QALY, whereas all the others used clinical outcome measures; and (iii) all studies were 'piggy-backed' (i.e. appendixed), thus no separate power analysis was performed for the economic evaluation study. That review concluded that few economic evaluations have been undertaken in the domain of stroke and recommended that QALYs should be used to quantify economic effects in stroke, especially as intangible costs such as psychosocial consequences play an important role (Evers et al, 2000).

## Measuring process as a proxy for outcome

As described below there is a substantial evidence base linking specific interventions to improved outcome. It is therefore reasonable to suppose that if an individual patient can be shown to have been managed appropriately, the chance of a better outcome will be higher. Where individual clinical services are attempting to evaluate the quality of care, compared to similar units, it is usually impossible to have sufficient numbers of patients to enable statistically significant differences in outcomes, such as death or disability, to be identified. This is likely to be the case even where there are important variations in the quality of care delivered. For this reason, audit of stroke care has to define the appropriate process of care and measure the degree of compliance with those standards (Rudd et al, 2001). The National Sentinel Audit of Stroke in the UK has shown that such an approach can differentiate between services and provide individual hospitals with data benchmarked against the national data. This can be used to inform service improvement (Rudd et al, 2001).

## Recommendation for future studies into stroke outcomes

Future studies into stroke outcomes should conduct longitudinal assessments, with a wide range of standardized measures covering all domains of stroke outcomes, at fixed time intervals in a population-based stroke cohort that includes all ages and stroke subtypes. The duration of follow-up should be long enough to determine changes in associations between performance-based measures and HRQOL over time, studies that examine differences in the HRQOL between men and women, and larger studies to confirm or refute the associations reported to date. In our opinion, a feasible time interval between each consecutive assessment in future studies on long-term outcomes would be 1 year. This interval would not only allow enough time for any change in handicap or HRQOL to be appreciated, but would also not be so long as to lose the perspectives of these domains. Furthermore, mortality rates should also be considered in conjunction with the prevalence rates of these domains, in order to address the potential confounding situation whereby a new intervention or process of care for stroke patients may enhance survival, but consequently yield more disabled and/or handicapped patients. The need for improved standards of long-term stroke care, including better community services (intermediate care), has received national recognition by the UK Government as reflected in its *National Service Framework for Older People* (Department of Health, 2001).

# Evidence for Stroke Rehabilitation Interventions

An intercollegiate working party for stroke has developed the National Clinical Guidelines for Stroke for England and Wales, under the auspices of the Royal College of Physicians of London (Wade and Rudd, 2000). These guidelines are based on a detailed review of the evidence for stroke rehabilitation interventions. Some of the important rehabilitation interventions will be discussed below.

## Service organization

The Stroke Unit Trialists' Collaboration (1997, 2000) conducted a meta-analysis of 19 studies ($n = 2060$ patients) and showed that stroke mortality and morbidity were significantly better in those stroke patients who were managed in specialist stroke units compared with those who were managed on general medical wards. Key features of such units should include:

1.  A geographically identified unit acting as a base, and as part of the inpatient service
2.  A coordinated multidisciplinary team
3.  Staff with specialist expertise in stroke and rehabilitation
4.  Educational programmes for staff, patients and carers
5.  Agreed protocols for common problems.

Two additional features of such units have been suggested in the guidelines although there is only grade C evidence for them:

6.  A neurovascular clinic for rapid assessment of transient ischaemic attack/minor stroke
7.  Access to brain and vascular imaging services.

## Specific rehabilitation interventions

Interventions have been tested to address problems in the following areas after stroke (Wade and Rudd, 2000):

*   psychological impairments: mood and cognitive disorders
*   communication: dysphasia, dysarthria and dyspraxia
*   motor impairment and spasticity
*   sensory impairment and pain, including shoulder pain
*   gait re-education
*   activities of daily living
*   equipment and adaptations.

Unfortunately, for many of these problems there is inadequate evidence to support specific treatments (Wade and Rudd, 2000). There are a few specific rehabilitation interventions for which there is grade A evidence. These are briefly outlined below.

## Psychological impairments: mood and cognitive disorders

There is much evidence on the prevalence of depression and cognitive impairment after stroke, but it is difficult to use the available evidence to guide specific treatment. The primary difficulty is in deciding whether a specific intervention is needed to improve the mood state and, if so, what intervention. Grade A evidence exists for the following situations:

- patients with severe, persistent or troublesome tearfulness (emotionalism) should be given antidepressant drug treatment, monitoring the frequency of crying to check effectiveness (Brown et al, 1998),
- patients in whom a depressive disorder has been diagnosed should be considered for a trial of antidepressant medication (Andersen et al, 1994), and
- patients with persistent visual neglect or visual field defects should be offered specific retraining strategies (Kalra et al, 1997).

## Communication: dysphasia, dysarthria and dyspraxia

Stroke can affect communication in different ways: dysarthria, dysphasia or articulatory dyspraxia. The patient may have subtle communication problems due to higher level language impairment associated with non-dominant hemisphere stroke. Accurate diagnosis is essential to guide and inform the team and the family. A speech and language therapist (SLT) is the most competent person to assess a patient with abnormal communication. There is evidence that if the patient has communication difficulties, the staff and relatives should be informed by the SLT of communication techniques appropriate to the impairment (Lyon et al, 1997). Also, where achievable goals can be identified and continuing progress demonstrated, patients with communication difficulties should be offered appropriate treatment, with monitoring of progress (Greener et al, 1999). Finally, for patients with long-term language difficulties, especially with reading, a period of reading retraining should be considered (Katz and Wertz, 1997).

## Motor impairment and spasticity

The aim of conventional therapeutic approaches is to increase physical independence through the facilitation of motor control and skill acquisition. Currently there is little evidence to support the effects of therapy on improving motor control (Wade and Rudd, 2000). There are additional techniques, such as biofeedback and functional electrical stimulation, that can be used as an adjunct to conventional therapy, but there is no convincing evidence to support these techniques.

Spasticity is a motor disorder characterized by a velocity-dependent increase in tonic stretch reflexes. In practice the management of spasticity may require several coordinated interventions, including physiotherapy and patient education. Despite being available for many years, and despite being widely promoted for and used in patients who have had a stroke, there is remarkably little evidence on the benefits or risks of using antispastic drugs (Wade and Rudd, 2000). There is minimal evidence concerning physical treatments. In contrast to the situation with systemic drugs or therapy, there is much more evidence relating to botulinum toxin (not all specific to stroke), presumably because it is expensive, it is effective, and it can be targeted without significant side effects (Hesse et al, 1998).

## Sensory impairment and pain, including shoulder pain

Patients who have suffered a stroke may experience pain of several types. Most of the pain is mechanical, arising from reduced mobility; some will come from premorbid diseases such as osteoarthritis; and a minority will be specific to stroke damage (central post-stroke pain). Chronic pain, especially central pain, may respond to tricyclic antidepressants and these should be tried sooner rather than later (Wiffen et al, 1999).

Transcutaneous electrical nerve stimulation (TENS) and acupuncture are both possible ways of giving sensory input. Their use is still being investigated; the mechanisms underlying benefit (if any) are unknown. Acupuncture and routine TENS for improving muscle control should only be used in the context of ongoing trials (Gosman-Hedstrom et al, 1998; Tekeoolu et al, 1998).

## Gait re-education

For the immobile patient, recovery of independent mobility is an important goal, and much therapy is devoted to gait re-education. Several of the topics considered earlier bear directly on mobility (e.g. botulinum toxin). There is evidence for gait re-education in the first weeks and months of rehabilitation. Treadmill training with partial (<40%) body weight support should be considered as an adjunct to conventional therapy in patients who are not walking at 3 months after stroke (Visintin et al, 1998).

## Activities of daily living

Much of stroke rehabilitation aims, directly or indirectly, to increase independence and ability in all activities of daily living (ADL), not only personal (e.g. dressing) but also domestic (e.g. cooking) and communal (e.g. shopping). All patients with difficulties in ADL should be assessed by an occupational therapist with specialist knowledge in neurological disability (Walker et al, 1999). Secondly, as mentioned earlier, patients with difficulties in ADL should be treated by a specialist multidisciplinary team (Stroke Unit Trialists' Collaboration, 1997, 2000).

## Equipment and adaptations

These can be divided into two main groups: personal aids and appliances.

### *Personal aids*

Small changes in an individual's local 'environment' can greatly increase independence: use of a wheelchair or walking stick; use of Velcro in place of buttons; use of adapted cutlery, etc. Many of these 'treatments' are so simple and small that it is unlikely that anyone will ever research into them. Nonetheless there are areas of controversy such as the use of walking aids and ankle-foot orthoses. It is acknowledged that walking aids and ankle-foot orthoses may benefit selected patients. Patients should be supplied as soon as possible with all aids and equipment needed (Mann et al, 1999).

### *Appliances*

This refers to any larger items or structural changes needed to alleviate the impact of a stroke-related impairment. Many patients have residual disability that can be helped by adapting their environment on a larger scale, for example, with stairlifts, hoists, perching stools or adaptations to buildings. Some of this equipment is supplied and funded by health services, a majority is supplied and funded by social services, some is funded by housing services, and some is not funded except by the patient and the family. Consequently there are major potential and actual problems in ensuring that the needs of patients are identified and then satisfied efficiently. There is grade A evidence that every patient who is at home or leaving hospital should be assessed fully to determine whether equipment or adaptations can increase safety or independence (Mann et al, 1999).

## Conclusions

The ultimate aim of stroke research and rehabilitation after stroke is to reduce impairment, disability and handicap and to enhance the quality of life. While our understanding of HRQOL of stroke patients is improving, our methods of altering it are still lagging behind. Current short-term trials of leisure therapy are addressing the issue of minimizing handicap even in the most disabled patients, especially in the area of occupation handicap (Gladman et al, 1996). A recent multicentre randomized controlled trial of leisure therapy and conventional occupational therapy in 466 patients reported that those who had leisure therapy showed a trend towards better albeit non-significant HRQOL and extended ADL scores compared with conventional occupational therapy at 6 and 12 months after stroke (Parker et al, 2001). Other short-term studies (Walker et al, 1999) have also reported on the benefits of occupational therapy for selected stroke cohorts, but long-term trials are required to capture their effects on long-term outcomes.

Future interventional studies in stroke should also be long enough to determine whether the effect of an intervention is longstanding. There are few randomized controlled trials (RCTs) that have examined the longer-term effects of interventions in stroke. Indredavik et al (1998) reported that treatment in stroke units was associated with better survival, functional outcome, less handicap and better quality of life compared with treatment in general medical wards up to 5 years after stroke. Carotid endarterectomy for symptomatic patients with 70–99% stenosis was shown to be efficacious for up to 3 years after the intervention in terms of ipsilateral stroke and further carotid artery stenosis and/or occlusion (Paciaroni et al, 2000). Dorman et al (1997) looked at long-term HRQOL using SF-36 and EuroQol on subjects recruited in the International Stroke Trial, but only compared the two HRQOL instruments. That study did not explore the effect of the interventions (i.e. use of aspirin and/or heparin after acute stroke) on HRQOL. Similar RCTs should be designed in future to capture broader, longer-term outcomes of various stroke interventions.

# References

Andersen G, Vestergaard K, Lauritsen L (1994) Effective treatment of post-stroke depression with the selective serotonin re-uptake inhibitor citalopram. *Stroke* **25**: 1099–104.

Bowling A (1995) *Measuring Disease: A Review of Disease-Specific Quality of Life Measurement Scales.* Open University Press, Buckingham.

Brown KW, Sloan RL, Pentland B (1998) Fluoxetine as a treatment for post-stroke emotionalism. *Acta Psychiatrica Scandinavia* **98**: 455–8.

Clarke PJ, Black SE, Badley EM, Lawrence JM, Williams JI (1999) Handicap in stroke survivors. *Disability and Rehabilitation* **21**: 116–23.

Department of Health (1993) Secretary of State for Health. *The Health of the Nation. Key Area Handbook: Coronary Heart Disease and Stroke,* 65. HMSO, London.

Department of Health (2001) *National Service Framework for Older People.* DoH, London (http://www.doh.gov.uk/nsf/olderpeople.htm).

Deyo RA, Carter WB (1992) Strategies for improving and expanding the application of health status measures in clinical settings. *Medical Care* **30**(Suppl 5): S176–S186, S196–S209.

Dijkerman HC, Wood VA, Hewer RL (1996) Long-term outcome after discharge from a stroke rehabilitation unit. *Journal of the Royal College of Physicians London* **30**: 538–46.

Donabedian A (1980) *Exploration in Quality Assessment and Monitoring, Vol 1. The Definition of Quality and Approaches to its Assessment.* Health Administration Press, Ann Arbor, Michigan.

Dorman P, Slattery JM, Farrell B, Dennis MS, Sandercock PA, and the United Kingdom Collaborators in the International Stroke Trial (1997) A randomised comparison of the EuroQol and SF-36 after stroke. *British Medical Journal* **315**: 461.

Dorman P, Dennis M, Sandercock P (2000) Are the modified "simple questions" a valid and reliable measure of health related quality of life after stroke? *Journal of Neurology Neurosurgery and Psychiatry* **69**: 487–93.

Duckworth D (1983) The classification and measurement of disablement. DHSS/HMSO, London.

Duncan PW, Samsa GP, Weinberger M et al (1997) Health status of individuals with mild stroke. *Stroke* **28**: 740–5.

Ebrahim S (1990) *Clinical Epidemiology of Stroke.* Oxford University Press, Oxford.

Evers SM, Ament AJ, Blaauw G (2000) Economic evaluation in stroke research: a systematic review. *Stroke* **31**: 1046–53.

Gladman JRF, Barer D, Langhorne P (1996) Specialist rehabilitation after stroke. *British Medical Journal* **312**: 1623–4.

Gold MR, Siegel JE, Russell LB, Weinstein MC (1996) *Cost-effectiveness in Health, and Medicine.* Oxford University Press, New York.

Gosman-Hedstrom G, Claesson L, Klingenstierna U et al (1998) Effects of acupuncture treatment on daily life activities and quality of life: a controlled prospective and randomised study of acute stroke patients. *Stroke* **29**: 2100–8.

Greener J, Enderby P, Whurr R (1999) Speech and language therapy for aphasia following stroke (Cochrane Review). In: *The Cochrane Library* Issue 4. Update Software, Oxford.

Greer S (1984) The psychological dimension in cancer treatment. *Social Science and Medicine* **18**: 345–9.

Hankey GJ, Jamrozik K, Broadhurst RJ et al (2000) Five-year survival after first-ever stroke and related prognostic factors in the Perth Community Stroke Study. *Stroke* **31**: 2080–6.

Harwood RH, Gompertz P, Ebrahim S (1994) Handicap one year after a stroke: validity of a new scale. *Journal of Neurology Neurosurgery and Psychiatry* **57**: 825–9.

Harwood RH, Gompertz P, Pound P, Ebrahim S (1997) Determinants of handicap 1 and 3 years after a stroke. *Disability and Rehabilitation* **19**: 205–11.

Hesse S, Reiter F, Konrad M, Jahnke MT (1998) Botulinum toxin type A and short-term electrical stimulation in the treatment of upper limb flexor spasticity after stroke: a randomised, double-blind, placebo-controlled trial. *Clinical Rehabilitation* **12**: 381–8.

Higginson IJ, Carr AJ (2001) Using quality of life measures in the clinical setting. *British Medical Journal* **322**: 1297–300.

Indredavik B, Bakke F, Slordahl SA, Rokseth R, Haheim LL (1998) Stroke unit treatment improves long-term quality of life: a randomized controlled trial. *Stroke* **29**: 895–9.

Kalra L, Perez I, Gupta S, Wittink M (1997) The influence of visual neglect on stroke rehabilitation. *Stroke* **28**: 1386–91.

Kaplan RM (1995) Quality of life measures. In: Karloy P, ed. *Measurement Strategies in Health Psychology*. John Wiley, New York.

Katz RC, Wertz RT (1997) The efficacy of computer-provided reading treatment for chronic aphasic adults. *Journal of Speech, Language and Hearing Research* **40**: 493–507.

Lindley RI, Waddell F, Livingstone M et al (1994) Can simple questions assess outcome after stroke? *Cerebrovascular Diseases* **4**: 314–24.

Long AF (1995) Clarifying and identifying the desired outcomes of an intervention: the case of stroke. *Outcomes Briefing* **5**: 10–12.

Lyon JG, Cariski D, Keisler L et al (1997) Communication partners: enhancing participation in life and communication for adults with aphasia in natural settings. *Aphasiology* **11**: 693–708.

McKevitt C, Dundas R, Wolfe C (2001) European BIOMED II Study of Stroke Care Group. Two simple questions to assess outcome after stroke: a European study. *Stroke* **32**: 681–6.

Mann WC, Ottenbacher KJ, Fraas L et al (1999) Effectiveness of assistive technology and environmental interventions in maintaining independence and reducing home care costs for the elderly. *Archives of Family Medicine* **8**: 210–17.

Martin J, White A, Meltzer H (1989) *Office of Population Censuses and Surveys. Disabled Adults: Services, Transport and Employment.* Report 4, Disability in Great Britain. HMSO, London.

Mayo NE, Wood-Dauphinee S, Ahmed S et al (1999) Disablement following stroke. *Disability and Rehabilitation* **21**: 258–68.

Murray CJ, Lopez AD (1997) Mortality by cause for eight regions of the world: Global Burden of Disease Study. *Lancet* **349**: 1269–76.

Office of National Statistics (1997) Series DH, 2 no. 24. *Mortality Statistics: Causes.* England and Wales. HMSO, London.

Paciaroni M, Eliasziw M, Sharpe BL et al (2000) Long-term clinical and angiographic outcomes in symptomatic patients with 70% to 99% carotid artery stenosis. *Stroke* **31**: 2037–42.

Parker CJ, Gladman JR, Drummond AE et al (2001) A multicentre randomized controlled trial of leisure therapy and conventional occupational therapy after stroke. TOTAL Study Group. Trial of Occupational Therapy and Leisure. *Clinical Rehabilitation* **15**: 42–52.

Patel M, McKevitt C, Tilling K, Rudd AG, Wolfe CDA (2001) Multidimensional longer-term stroke outcomes. *Expert Review of Pharmacoeconomics and Outcomes Research* **1**: 109–17.

Patrick DL, Deyo RA (1989) Generic and disease-specific measures in assessing health status and quality of life. *Medical Care* **27**: S217–S232.

Roberts L, Counsell C (1998) Assessment of clinical outcomes in acute stroke trials. *Stroke* **29**: 986–91.

Rudd AG, Irwin P, Lowe D, Rutledge Z, Pearson P (2001) National Clinical Audit. A tool for change. *Quality in Healthcare* **10**: 141–51.

Samuelsson M, Soderfeldt B, Olsson GB (1996) Functional outcome in patients with lacunar infarction. *Stroke* **27**: 842–6.

Seale C, Davies P (1987) Outcome measurement in stroke rehabilitation research. *International Disability Studies* **9**: 155–60.

Stojcevic N, Wilkinson P, Wolfe C (1996) Outcome measurement in stroke patients. In: Wolfe C, Rudd A, Beech R, eds. *Stroke Services & Research: An Overview, With Recommendations for Future Research,* 261–80. The Stroke Association, London.

Stroke Unit Trialists Collaboration (1997) How do stroke units improve patient outcomes? A collaborative systematic review of the randomized trials. *Stroke* **28**: 2139–44.

Stroke Unit Trialists' Collaboration (2000) Organised inpatient (stroke unit) care for stroke. *Cochrane Database Systematic Review* (2): CD000197.

Task Force on Stroke Impairment, Task Force on Stroke Disability, and Task Force on Stroke Handicap (1990) Symposium recommendations for methodology in stroke outcome research. *Stroke* **21**(Suppl 9): 1168–73.

Tekeoolu Y, Adak B, Goksoy T (1998) Effect of transcutaneous electrical nerve stimulation (TENS) on Barthel Activities of Daily Living (ADL) index score following stroke. *Clinical Rehabilitation* **12**: 277–80.

Tilley BC, Marler J, Geller NL et al (1996) Use of a global test for multiple outcomes in stroke trials with application to the National Institute of Neurological Disorders and t-PA Stroke Trial. *Stroke* **27**: 2136–42.

Visintin M, Barbeau H, Korner-Bitensky N, Mayo NE (1998) A new approach to retrain gait in stroke patients through body weight support and tread-mill stimulation. *Stroke* **29**: 1122–8.

Wade DT (1992) *Measurement in Neurological Rehabilitation.* Oxford University Press, Oxford.

Wade DT, Hewer RL (1987) Functional abilities after stroke: measurement, natural history and prognosis. *Journal of Neurology Neurosurgery and Psychiatry* **50**: 177–82.

Wade DT, Rudd AG and the intercollegiate working party for stroke (2000) National Clinical Guidelines for Stroke. *Royal College of Physicians of London* **34**: 131–3.

Walker MF, Gladman JR, Lincoln NB, Siemonsma P, Whiteley T (1999) Occupational therapy for stroke patients not admitted to hospital: a ran-domised controlled trial. *Lancet* **354**: 278–80.

Wiffen P, McQuay H, Carroll D et al (1999) Anticonvulsant drugs for acute and chronic pain (Cochrane Review). In: *The Cochrane Library*, Issue 3. Update Software, Oxford.

Wood P (1980) *International Classification of Impairments, Disabilities and Handicaps: A Manual of Classification Relating to the Consequences of Disease.* World Health Organization, Geneva.

World Health Organization (1999) *ICIDH-2: International Classification of Functioning and Disability.* (Beta-2 draft.) WHO, Geneva (www.who.int/icidh/).

# 6

# Service Delivery and Models of Care

*Lalit Kalra*

There is strong clinical evidence from meta-analysis of randomized controlled trials that stroke units reduce mortality, institutionalization and disability. Stroke care has several interdependent components, which include multidisciplinary care, specific interventions, physiological homeostasis, prevention of complications, assessment of rehabilitation needs, and early mobilization. Even with specialist support, such care cannot be replicated for acute patients on general medical wards. In view of the strength of evidence, stroke patients should be managed on stroke units by specialist stroke teams.

## Introduction

Stroke is the third commonest cause of death and the biggest cause of severe disability in Western countries (Bonita et al, 1995). Recent advances in neuroimaging and vascular imaging, understanding of pathophysiological mechanisms and treatments such as thrombolysis have transformed the way stroke is managed (Thomassen et al, 2003). There is now increased emphasis on early investigations and interventions, which require timely and coordinated input from several disciplines. Fundamental to providing this input effectively and efficiently is the concept of the stroke unit (Kidwell et al, 2003). Several studies have shown that such units improve quality of care as well as outcomes for the vast majority of stroke patients (Stroke Unit Trialists' Collaboration, 2000).

Although a stroke unit has been defined as 'a service provided on a discrete stroke ward or by a dedicated team of professionals working exclusively in the care of stroke patients' (Warlow et al, 1996), several different models exist in clinical practice:

1.  Stroke intensive care unit: where patients are admitted directly to a unit with intensive monitoring equipment for a short period of time.
2.  Acute stroke unit: patients admitted directly from the community in the early stages of stroke, remaining for a variable length of time prior to rehabilitation.
3.  Stroke rehabilitation unit: primarily concerned with rehabilitation, admitting patients from general wards or acute stroke units when medically stable.
4.  Combined acute and rehabilitation unit.
5.  Stroke team: which consults throughout the hospital wherever a stroke patient is admitted and provides continuity of specialist care.
6.  Domiciliary stroke care: where a team of specialists in rehabilitation supports patients at home without need for admission to hospital or after early discharge from hospital.

## Stroke Intensive Care Units (SICUs)

Stroke intensive care units (SICUs) are based on the principles of an intensive care unit and provide optimal care under intensive monitored conditions for 3–4 days after acute onset (Busse, 2003). Advantages of such units include the ability to provide specific aggressive pharmacological and surgical interventions under close supervision and to develop new therapeutic concepts based on physiological manipulation of factors that may affect cerebral blood flow and metabolism. Another objective of such units is to minimize neurological complications in order to reduce the amount of secondary damage to the brain. Core practices on such units include rapid normalization of oxygenation, blood volume, glucose and temperature; maintenance of blood pressure and high cardiac output; and continuous monitoring of intracranial pressure with early intervention.

The evidence for supporting intensive care units is relatively sparse, with only a few small randomized controlled trials being reported in the 1970s (Stroke Unit Trialists' Collaboration, 2000). These showed no difference in outcome, but patients managed on SICUs appeared to have fewer complications and quicker investigations. It is probable that newer studies may show benefit because of advances in acute stroke treatment. Such studies will prove hard to design and undertake.

## Acute Stroke Unit (ASU)

Acute stroke units (ASUs) are modelled on the lines of a high dependency unit. Core practices include early establishment of diagnosis, type and aetiology of stroke using a range of investigative techniques and institution of measures to reduce damage, which can be specific (e.g. thrombolysis) or generic (physiological monitoring) (Brown and Haley, 2002). Measures are undertaken to prevent stroke-related complications, treat comorbidity and prevent recurrence by appropriate and adequate secondary prevention. Factors associated with ASU care include increased use of oxygen, intravenous fluids and antipyretics; stabilization of blood glucose levels; prevention of aspiration; early nutrition and early mobilization. These are underpinned by teamwork and staff education on the specialist aspects of stroke management.

Evidence suggests that ASUs are highly effective in improving stroke outcome because of the existence of defined processes of integrated interdisciplinary care (Evans et al, 2001). Key factors responsible for this benefit include attention to physiological homeostasis, greater or earlier therapy input, attention to comorbidity, complications and secondary prevention and higher expectations of staff and patients. The individual contribution of each of these modalities is unknown and merits further research.

## Stroke Rehabilitation Units (SRUs)

Stroke rehabilitation units (SRUs) are the most researched and the most prevalent strategy for providing stroke care. Whilst recognizing the heterogeneity of SRU care, the Stroke Unit Trialists' Collaboration (SUTC) identified a number of key areas in which organized stroke care differed from general medical care (Stroke Unit Trialists' Collaboration, 1997). These include:

- multidisciplinary team care (including the integration of nurses into the team)
- physician and nursing interest in stroke
- earlier onset and increased physiotherapy and occupational therapy
- involvement of carers in rehabilitation.

In the 1980s to 1990s a number of randomized controlled trials suggested that organized rehabilitation offered advantages to patients with stroke, but many of these studies were too small to demonstrate a robust statistical benefit. A systematic review and meta-analysis of 19 trials (from Australia, North America and Europe) by the SUTC showed an odds reduction of 20% for death, 28% for death or institutionalization and 32% for death or dependency for SRU care over general medical ward care (Stroke Unit Trialists' Collaboration, 2000). The effect was independent of age and gender. Furthermore, although the majority of patients had strokes of moderate severity, patients with milder and more severe strokes also benefited. Since the review was published, follow-up data from two studies have been reported which show that the observed differences persist for many years (Indredavik et al, 1999; Lincoln et al, 2000).

## Stroke Team (ST)

It may not always be possible to admit all stroke patients to a specialist setting because of limited availability of facilities in certain settings. The concept of the stroke team was suggested for such situations where patients continue to remain on general wards under the care of admitting physicians (Wood-Dauphinee et al, 1984). However, they are assessed by a specialist team who provide a plan of management based on standardized evidence-based guidelines for care. The care plan is implemented by generic ward teams but with regular advice from the specialist team. Core practices include standardized diagnostic evaluation, advice on prevention of complications, secondary prevention and early mobilization with clearly defined goals for rehabilitation. Evidence shows that despite the specialist input, patients on general medical wards are twice as likely to die or need care in an institution as those on a combined acute and rehabilitation stroke unit (Figure 6.1) (Kalra et al, 2000).

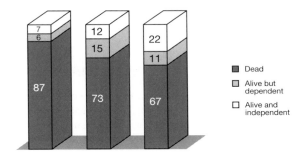

**Figure 6.1** Outcome at 1 year with different strategies of stroke care. Difference per 100 patients treated: stroke unit vs domicillary care: 14 more alive and independent (NNT = 7); stroke unit vs stroke team: 20 more alive and independent (NNT = 5).
(NNT, number needed to treat.)

## Domiciliary Stroke Care

In some European countries up to 50% of stroke patients are not admitted to hospital (Shah and Harwood, 1999). Although there are theoretical advantages to rehabilitation in a familiar environment, acute stroke patients appear to do worse. Moderately severe acute stroke patients randomly assigned to specialist management at home were significantly more likely to die or be institutionalized than those on a stroke unit and a third had to be admitted to hospital in the first 2 weeks (Kalra et al, 2000). This supports the WHO Pan-European Consensus on Stroke Care, which advocates early hospital-based management (Aboderin and Venables, 1996).

An alternative option to hospital-based care is the concept of prompt supported discharge that commences as soon as the patient is medically stable enough to leave hospital and comprises home-based rehabilitation and medical services (Outpatient Service Trialists, 2003). Several early randomized controlled trials suggest that early supported discharge reduced length of stay without any detrimental (or beneficial) effect on motor, functional or social outcomes (Rudd et al, 1997; Anderson et al, 2000). The implications were that although prompt discharge and home care was more economical than hospital care, there were no benefits to patients. More recent studies have challenged this view and shown that prompt discharge combined with home rehabilitation appeared to translate motor and functional gains that occur through natural recovery and rehabilitation into a greater degree of higher level function and satisfaction with community reintegration, and these in turn were translated into a better physical health. Providing care at home was no more (or less) expensive for those with greater functional limitation than for those with lesser disability (Mayo et al, 2000; Anderson et al, 2002). Caregivers of patients who receive early supported discharge showed lower caregiver burden, suggesting that early supported discharge provided a cost-effective alternative to hospital care for persons recovering from stroke and their families (Anderson et al, 2002; Teng et al, 2003).

## Are Stroke Units Cost-effective?

There have been no published studies directly comparing the costs of a stroke unit with care on general medical wards. The majority of hospital costs associated with stroke appear to be related to length of inpatient stay and it is likely that stroke units reduce costs of hospital care by reducing the length of hospital stay (Bergman et al, 1995). However, the real cost of a stroke unit may be greater than alternate strategies of offering stroke care. Analysis of cost data using a societal perspective from a published randomized controlled study (Kalra et al, 2000) showed mean health and social care costs over 12 months of £11,450 for stroke unit, £9,527 for stroke team and £6,840 for domiciliary care. More than half the costs were for the initial episode of care, although institutionalization dominated follow-up costs. The inclusion of informal care increases costs considerably (Dewey et al, 2001). It appears that stroke units improve health outcomes significantly, but they come at a higher cost. More importantly, if all stroke patients are to be managed on stroke units, there will be additional costs of infrastructure and training, especially for medical and nursing staff. At present, physicians and nurses who look after stroke patients come from a variety of backgrounds including general medicine, neurology, geriatric medicine and rehabilitation. Stroke physicians and nurses need a wide range of clinical abilities, as the management of stroke requires expertise in prevention, diagnosis, acute treatment and rehabilitation (Bath et al, 1997). This presents a particular challenge, as training which covers all aspects of stroke care is not provided within any of the existing specialities. Hence, choices need to be made by health services and society regarding how much we are prepared to invest in and pay for improvements in outcomes in stroke, a disorder which affects mostly older individuals and, until recently, was characterized by patient and professional nihilism.

## Conclusion

Care on a stroke unit is associated with reduced mortality, institutionalization and disability for patients with a wide range of stroke severity. The evidence in favour of stroke unit treatment compares favourably with other interventions that would be considered essential management. There are several different ways in which organized stroke care can be delivered, and patient needs, organizational aspects or specific medical interventions are likely to dictate the strategy most likely to benefit the majority of patients in the setting. Regardless of the way stroke care is organized, it is unacceptable to offer non-specialist management to patients with stroke in the era of evidence-based medicine.

## References

Aboderin I, Venables G (1996) Stroke management in Europe. Pan European Consensus Meeting on Stroke Management. *Journal of Internal Medicine* **240**: 173–80.

Anderson C, Rubenbach S, Mhurchu CN, Clark M, Spencer C, Winsor A (2000) Home or hospital for stroke rehabilitation? Results of a randomised controlled trial I: health outcomes at 6 months. *Stroke* **31**:1024–31.

Anderson C, Ni Mhurchu C, Brown PM, Carter K (2002) Stroke rehabilitation services to accelerate hospital discharge and provide home-based care: an overview and cost analysis. *Pharmacoeconomics* **20**: 537–52.

Bath P, Lees K, Dennis M et al (1997) Should stroke medicine be a separate subspecialty? *British Medical Journal* **315**: 1167–8.

Bergman L, van der Meulen JHP, Limburg M, Habbedema JDF (1995) Costs of medical care after first-ever stroke in the Netherlands. *Stroke* **26**: 1830–6.

Bonita R, Steward A, Beaglehole R (1995) International trends in stroke mortality. *Stroke* **21**: 989–92.

Brown DL, Haley EC (2002) Post-emergency department management of stroke. *Emergency Medicine Clinics of North America* **20**: 687–702.

Busse O (2003) Stroke units and stroke services in Germany. *Cerebrovascular Diseases* **15** (Suppl 1): 8–10.

Dewey HM, Thrift AG, Mihalopoulos C et al (2001) Cost of stroke in Australia from a societal perspective: results from the North East Melbourne Stroke Incidence Study (NEMESIS). *Stroke* **32**: 2409–16.

Evans A, Perez I, Harraf F et al (2001) Can differences in management processes explain different outcomes between stroke unit and stroke-team care? *Lancet* **358**: 1586–92.

Indredavik B, Bakke F, Slørdahl SA, Rokseth R, Haheim LL (1999) Stroke unit treatment. 10-year follow-up. *Stroke* **30**: 1524–7.

Kalra L, Evans A, Perez I, Knapp M, Donaldson N, Swift CG (2000) Alternative strategies for stroke care: a prospective randomised controlled trial. *Lancet* **356**: 894–9.

Kidwell CS, Shephard T, Tonn S et al (2003) Establishment of primary stroke centers: a survey of physician attitudes and hospital resources. *Neurology* **60**: 1452–6.

Lincoln NB, Husbands S, Trescoli C, Drummond AER, Gladman JRF, Berman P (2000) Five year follow up of a randomised controlled trial of a stroke rehabilitation unit. *British Medical Journal* **320**: 549.

Mayo NE, Wood-Dauphinee S, Côté R et al (2000) There's no place like home. An evaluation of early supported discharge for stroke. *Stroke* **31**: 1016–23.

Outpatient Service Trialists (2003) Therapy-based rehabilitation services for stroke patients at home. *Cochrane Database Systematic Review* (1): CD002925.

Rudd AG, Wolfe CDA, Tilling K, Beech R (1997) Randomised controlled trial to evaluate early discharge scheme for patients with stroke. *British Medical Journal* **315**: 1039–44.

Shah E, Harwood R (1999) Acute management: admission to hospital. In: *Stroke: epidemiology, evidence and clinical practice*, 2nd edn. Oxford University Press, Oxford.

Stroke Unit Trialists' Collaboration (1997) How do stroke units improve patient outcomes? A collaborative systematic review of the randomized trials. *Stroke* **28**: 2139–44.

Stroke Unit Trialists' Collaboration (2000) Organised inpatient (stroke unit) care for stroke. *Cochrane Database Systematic Review* (2): CD000197.

Teng J, Mayo NE, Latimer E et al (2003) Costs and caregiver consequences of early supported discharge for stroke patients. *Stroke* **34**: 528–36.

Thomassen L, Brainin M, Demarin V, Grond M, Toni D, Venables GS (2003) Acute stroke treatment in Europe: a questionnaire-based survey on behalf of the EFNSTask Force on acute neurological stroke care. *European Journal of Neurology* **10**: 199–204.

Warlow CP, Dennis MS, van Gijn J et al (1996) *Stroke. A practical guide to management*, 608–12. Blackwell, London.

Wood-Dauphinee S, Shapiro S, Bass E et al (1984) A randomized trial of team care following stroke. *Stroke* **15**: 864–72.

# Index